PROSTATE CANCER PREVENTION AND WHOLISTIC TREATMENT

NATURAL NON-TOXIC CHEMOTHERAPY FOR PROSTATE CANCER

BY

Dr. Brian K. Bailey

© 2016

The health information in this book is meant to be used by the reader and his or her primary care physician

These statements have not been evaluated by the Food and Drug Administration.

These products are not intended to diagnose, treat, cure, or prevent any disease.

**ISBN-13:
978-1533085122**

**ISBN-10:
1533085129**

$19.99 USA

DEDICATION

To my loving supportive wife, Cynthia whose
unconditional love I can rely on.
To my five children, four of which are boys, Jeremy,
Jared, Jonathan, Jeffery and daughter, Jennifer. I hope
they follow the advice herein. Also, to my 11
grandchildren

CONTENTS

ACKNOWLEDGMENTS

I greatly appreciate all the information and research at Life Extension especially: Life Extension Magazine December 2013 A Natural Arsenal for Prostate Cancer Prevention By Michael Downey. This article gave me ground work for research about the nutrients that affect the prostate.

I am also very thankful to http://www.ncbi.nlm.nih.gov/ Their databases are wonderful for research.

1 NUTRIENTS FOR PROSTATE CANCER PREVENTION AND ERADICATION

Not too many years ago men who had prostate cancer were castrated, had their testes surgically removed. Now, that is done chemically. Currently this is the first line treatment. This is done thinking that testosterone is the enemy. All this treatment does, is buy time. In a year or so, androgen insensitive cancer cells will take over. Poisonous chemotherapy with very expensive drugs is the next treatment. So, we go from no testosterone causing depression, lack of energy, loss of libido, muscle atrophy leading to weakness and increased risk of death for all causes to chemotherapy with its side effects.

They are still treating men with high doses of estrogen turning men into women with breasts. The thinking was estrogen opposes testosterone, wrong. Unbalanced estrogen is the enemy. It also causes cardiovascular disease when unbalanced with progesterone or testosterone.

A 15-year study published in the July 19, 2012 issue of the *New England Journal of Medicine* found that prostate cancer survival rates were the same whether men with early-stage disease were randomly assigned to have surgery or to a "watchful waiting" group. Over the 15 years that they were followed, a total of 52 men (about 7 percent of the 731 who participated) died of their cancer, but the researchers reported that there was no statistical difference between the two groups. (Some of the men in the study died from other causes, but here, too there was no statistical difference between the two groups.). **The men who had surgery had no survival advantage over those in the watchful waiting group.**

Prostate cancer is the second highest cancer-related cause of death. Nowadays, the aim of treatments is to decrease the effects of androgens on this organ. Unfortunately, over time, patients develop an androgen-independent cancer with a fatal outcome. The main features of late stage prostate cancer are an increased cell proliferation and apoptosis (cell suicide) resistance.

One in three American men have prostate cancer by age 50. Thirty-eight thousand have their prostates removed by surgery or radiation, and 40,000 men die from prostate cancer each year.

Autopsy evidence indicates that prostate cancer is histologically evident in up to 34% of men aged 40 to 49 and up to 70% of men aged 80 and older.

Is this inevitable? Is this, and enlarged prostates in 80% of American men just part of aging for the male? No, most of the world has no significant prostate problems. What are we doing to cause this epidemic?

Forty years ago experimenters showed that cancer cells could be caused to revert to normal, by changing their environment. This book will explain how to change cellular environment to prevent and eradicate cancer.

Many years ago, a pathologist said that he had been able to find diagnosable cancer somewhere in the body of every person over the age of 50 that he had autopsied. If everyone has cancer by the age of 50, that means that cancer is harmless for most people, and that small cancers might frequently appear, and be spontaneously removed as part of the body's regular house-cleaning.

In 1927, Bernstein and Elias found that rats eating a fat free diet had almost no spontaneous cancer, and many studies since then in animals and people have shown a close association between polyunsaturated fatty acids and cancer. Polyunsaturated fatty acids are highly reactive and cause mutations leading to cancer.

Eliminating polyunsaturated fats (PUFA) from the diet is essential if these carcinogenic changes are to be arrested. Aspirin and salicylic acid can block many of the carcinogenic effects of the PUFA. Saturated fats have a variety of anti-inflammatory and anticancer actions. Some of those effects are direct, others are the result of blocking the toxic effects of PUFA. Keeping the stored unsaturated fats from circulating in the blood is helpful, since it takes years to eliminate them from the tissues after the diet has changed.

Naloxone or naltrexone, which blocks the actions of the endorphins and morphine, is being used to inhibit the growth of various kinds of cancer, including breast cancer and prostate cancer. Leptin (which is promoted by estrogen) is a hormone produced by fat cells, and it, like estrogen, activates the POMC-related endorphin stress system. The endorphins activate histamine, another promoter of inflammation and cell division.

2 Tracking the Culprit

Why does prostate cancer occur so often in aging men? Consider the changes in testicular hormone production as men age:

1. Testosterone levels fall;

2. More testosterone is changed (by 5-alpha-reductase enzyme) to dihydrotestosterone (DHT), stimulating prostate growth and cancer;

3. Progesterone levels fall. Progesterone is vital to good health in men. It is the primary precursor of our adrenal cortical hormones and testosterone. Men synthesize progesterone in smaller amounts than women do but it is still vital. Since progesterone is a potent inhibitor of 5-alpha-reductase, the decline of progesterone in aging males plays a role in increasing the conversion rate of testosterone to DHT. More information about estrogen and progesterone later.

4. Estradiol (an estrogen) increases. Testosterone is a direct antagonist of estradiol. Both the fall in testosterone and the shift from testosterone to DHT allows increased effect of estradiol. Male estradiol levels are equivalent to or greater than that of postmenopausal females, but normally estradiol's effects are suppressed (antagonized) by the male's

greater production of testosterone. Estradiol is the culprit (along with DHT) in prostate growth. Also, IGF-1

Carcinogenesis. 2013 Sep;34(9):2017-23. doi: 10.1093/carcin/bgt156. Epub 2013 May 8.

High circulating estrogens and selective expression of ERβ in prostate tumors of Americans: implications for racial disparity of prostate cancer.

In comparison with normal age-matched subjects, circulating E2 levels were significantly elevated in all PCa patients.

Avoid xenoestrogens (from many plastics including can liners and pesticides).

Diet's role

Vegan Men: More Testosterone But Less Cancer, Written by: Michael Greger M.D. on February 12th, 2013

Excerpts:

Just a few days of walking and eating whole healthy plant foods and our IGF-1 levels drop low enough to reverse cancer cell growth.

After 11 days, it gets better. People eating plant-based foods 14 years have half the IGF-1 in their bodies, and more than twice the IGF binding protein than those on the Standard American Diet (SAD).

A study was done to determine whether a plant-based diet is associated with a lower circulating level of IGF-1 compared with a meat-eating or lacto-ovo-vegetarian diet, and this is what they found. Only the vegans had significantly lower levels. And the same relationship found with IGF-binding capacity. Only the vegans were significantly able to bind up excess IGF-1 in their blood streams.

The blood of those on a Standard American Diet (S.A.D.) fights cancer, but the blood of those on vegan diets fights about 8 times better. The blood circulating within the bodies of vegans appears to have nearly eight times the stopping power when it comes to cancer cell growth. That was after maintaining a plant-based diet for a year though. Studies on breast cancer showed the power of eating plants for just two weeks.

Dean Ornish, MD cardiologist conquered the number one killer, heart disease, now he's moved on to trying to reverse killer number 2, cancer.

PSA levels are typically what's used to follow the progression of prostate cancer. In the Standard American Diet group they got worse, in the vegan diet group they got better. No surgery, no chemotherapy, no radiation—they just started getting better.

To figure out what was going on, they took blood from each group and dripped their blood on prostate cancer cells in a petri dish to see what affect the dietary change had. The blood of the standard diet patients did reduce the cancer cell growth rates by about 10%. Their bodies, their immune systems were doing what they could to beat back the cancer. The blood of people on a vegan diet, though, knocked the cancer growth down 70%. Eating a plant-based diet made their bloodstream eight times less hospitable to cancer.

Ornish's two year follow up showed a significant number of the standard diet group were forced to go into surgery for what's called a radical prostatectomy, which often leads to urinary incontinence and impotence in 60% of men coming out of surgery. But not a single one of the men on the plant-based diet had to go to surgery.

Just a few things have been found associated with significantly increased risk for the disease: refined grains, like white bread, eggs, and poultry, which appeared even worse than red meat or desserts!

Top cancer fighting foods: Spinach and beets works against all types of cancer. Garlic completely 100% stopped cancer growth in 7 out of the 8 tumor lines. "the inclusion of cruciferous and allium vegetables in the diet is essential for effective dietary-based chemopreventive strategies."

Almonds appear twice as protective as lesser nuts, halving cancer cell growth at only half the dose, but these three are the winners, causing a dramatic drop in cancer proliferation at just tiny doses: walnuts and pecans, number three is peanuts.

A Low Methionine Diet May Help Starve Cancer Cells

Written by: Michael Greger M.D. on July 8th, 2014

Forty years ago, a landmark paper was published showing for the first time that many human cancers have what's called "absolute methionine dependency," meaning that if we try to grow cells in a Petri dish without giving them the amino acid methionine, normal cells thrive, but without methionine, cancer cells die. Normal breast cells grow no matter what, with or without methionine, but cancer cells need that added methionine to grow.

What does cancer do with the methionine? Tumors use it to generate gaseous sulfur-containing compounds that, interestingly, can be detected by specially trained diagnostic dogs. There are mole-sniffing dogs that can pick out skin cancer. There are breath-sniffing dogs that can pick out people with lung cancer. Pee-sniffing dogs that can diagnose bladder cancer and—you guessed it—fart-sniffing dogs for colorectal cancer. Doctors can now bring their lab to the lab!

It gives a whole new meaning to the term "petSCAN ." :)

Methionine dependency is not just present in cancer cell lines in a Petri dish. Fresh tumors taken from patients show that many cancers appear to have a biochemical defect that makes them dependent on methionine, including some tumors of the colon, breast, ovary, prostate, and skin. Pharmaceutical companies are fighting to be the first to come out with a drug that decreases methionine levels. But since methionine is sourced mainly from food, a better strategy may be to lower methionine levels by lowering methionine intake, eliminating high methionine foods to control cancer growth as well as improve our lifespan.

Here's the thinking: smoking cessation, consumption of DIETS rich in plants, and other lifestyle measures can prevent the majority of cancers. Unfortunately, people don't do them, and as a result hundreds of thousands of Americans develop metastatic cancer each year. Chemotherapy cures only a few types of metastatic cancer. Unfortunately, the vast majority of common metastatic cancers, such as breast, prostate, colon, and lung, are lethal. We therefore desperately need novel treatment strategies for metastatic cancer, and dietary methionine restriction may be one such strategy.

So, where is methionine found? Chicken and fish have the highest levels. Milk, red meat, and eggs have less, but if we really want to stick with lower methionine foods, fruits, nuts, veggies, grains, and beans are the best. In other words, "In humans, methionine restriction may be achieved using a predominately vegan DIET ."

More information about diet, is found on page 110

Testosterone's role

In 1995, Jarow et al. found no correlation between PSA and serum testosterone variations within the normal physiologic range and concluded that serum testosterone levels do not significantly alter the accuracy of PSA for the detection, staging and monitoring of prostate cancer. Moreover, data collected from more than 1500 men in the Massachusetts Male Aging Study, showed no significant relationship between prostate cancer risk and serum androgen concentrations.

In a recent (2008) collaborative analysis of 18 prospective studies (including 3886 men with prostate cancer and 6438 control participants), the investigators found no association between the risk of prostate cancer and 'endogenous' serum concentrations of testosterone (total and free), dihydrotestosterone and other serum androgens. In the same year, Mearini et al. (2008) reported that endogenous levels of testosterone were significantly lower in patients with prostate cancer (vs BPH) and that low testosterone levels were an independent predictor of advanced (vs organ-confined) disease. Most recently, Rhoden et al. (2008) discovered that a low (<1.8) testosterone-to-PSA ratio predicted prostate cancer on biopsy in symptomatic hypogonadal men with a PSA 4 ng ml before testosterone therapy.

The study by Muller et al provides the ultimate evidence disproving the androgen hypothesis (testosterone increases prostate cancer) and supporting the saturation model (higher testosterone level have no effect on prostate cancer).

There are multiple reports that suggest increased Prostate cancer risk with lower testosterone. Additionally, prostate cancer rates declined at the upper end of serum testosterone

Additional evidence supporting the androgen receptor saturation hypothesis was recently provided by Marks et al. (2006) who, in landmark randomized, double-blind, placebo-controlled trial analyzed prostate tissue concentrations of the principal androgens of the prostate (testosterone and dihydrotestosterone) following six months of parenteral TRT in hypogonadal patients. Despite significant increases in serum testosterone concentrations to normal physiologic levels, researchers identified no significant changes in serum PSA, prostate tissue testosterone and dihydrotestosterone concentrations, or prostate cancer biomarkers and gene expression within the prostate tissue itself.

J Urol. 2011 Apr;185(4):1256-60. doi: 10.1016/j.juro.2010.11.084. Epub 2011 Feb 22.

Testosterone therapy in men with untreated prostate cancer.

CONCLUSIONS:

Testosterone therapy in men with untreated prostate cancer was not associated with prostate cancer progression in the short to medium term. These results are consistent with the saturation model, ie maximal prostate cancer growth is achieved at low androgen concentrations. The longstanding prohibition against testosterone therapy in men with untreated or low risk prostate cancer or treated prostate cancer without evidence of metastatic or recurrent disease merits reevaluation.

J Steroid Biochem Mol Biol. 2006 Dec;102(1-5):261-6.

Prostate cancer risk in testosterone-treated men.

Data from all published prospective studies on circulating level of total and free testosterone **do not** support the hypothesis that high levels of circulating androgens are associated with an increased risk of prostate cancer. A study on a large prospective cohort of 10,049 men, contributes to the gathering evidence that the long standing "androgen hypothesis" of increasing risk with increasing androgen levels can be **rejected**, suggesting instead that **high levels** within the reference range of androgens, estrogens and adrenal androgens **decrease aggressive prostate cancer risk.** Indeed, **high-grade prostate cancer has been associated with low plasma level of testosterone**. Furthermore, pre-treatment total testosterone was an independent predictor of extraprostatic disease in patients with localized prostate cancer; as testosterone **decreases**, patients have an increased likelihood of non-organ confined disease and low serum testosterone levels are associated with positive surgical margins (metastasis) in radical retropubic prostatectomy.

Asian J Androl. 2014 Nov-Dec;16(6):864-8. doi: 10.4103/1008-682X.129132.

Physiological normal levels of androgen inhibit proliferation of prostate cancer cells in vitro.

For more than 70 years, it has been believed that a severe reduction of serum androgen levels caused regression of prostate cancer (PCa) and that increasing androgen levels enhanced growth of PCa. Both of the optimal androgen levels are within the adult men's physiological low range (<2.4 ng ml^{-1}). At **lower concentrations** than the optimal androgen level, promoted the proliferation of PCa cells. However, at the higher concentrations, resulted in a dose-dependent proliferative inhibition. We conclude that physiologically normal levels of androgen inhibit the proliferation of PCa cells in vitro. However, at very low levels androgens are essential for initial growth of PCa cells.

Progesterone's role

The male hormone, testosterone, is antagonist to estradiol. Testosterone prevents estradiol from causing prostate cancer by destroying the prostate cancer cells it stimulates.

Testosterone does NOT cause prostate cancer. If this were true 19 and 20 year old males would be developing prostate cancer as these are the individuals with the highest levels. This is obviously not the case. Males also produce progesterone, although about half as much as females do. The progesterone prevents the body from converting testosterone to di-hydro testosterone.

It does this by inhibiting the enzyme 5-alpha reductase. Progesterone inhibits 5-alpha reductase far more effectively than Proscar™ and Saw Palmetto which are the more standard agents employed in traditional and natural medicine.

As a male ages, his progesterone level decreases just like it does in women. In women this decease occurs about the age of 35 and men about ten years later. When progesterone levels decrease, the male's 5-alpha reductase converts the testosterone to di-hydro testosterone which is useless at removing the prostate cancer cells that estradiol stimulates. Estradiol also stimulates the enlargement of the prostate. This allows the prostate gland to swell and enlarge and in many cases transform into prostate cancer.

The prostate is embryologically similar to the female uterus.

Estradiol turns on the bcl-2 gene that promotes carcinogenic changes. Progesterone is the counter balance, progesterone turns on the guardian angel P-53 gene that causes cell apoptosis (suicide) in cells that become cancer. An interesting side note is that Benzo[a]pyrene a component of tobacco smoke turns this gene off. This results in increased cancer of all types in smokers.

3. SCREENING

Cochrane Database Syst Rev. 2013 Jan 31;1:CD004720. doi: 10.1002/14651858.CD004720.pub3.

Screening for prostate cancer.

Prostate cancer screening did not significantly decrease prostate cancer-specific mortality in a combined meta-analysis of five RCTs. Only one study (ERSPC) reported a 21% significant reduction of prostate cancer-specific mortality in a pre-specified subgroup of men aged 55 to 69 years. Pooled data currently demonstrates no significant reduction in prostate cancer-specific and overall mortality. Harms associated with PSA-based screening and subsequent diagnostic evaluations are frequent, and moderate in severity. Over diagnosis and overtreatment are common and are associated with treatment-related harms. Men should be informed of this and the demonstrated adverse effects when they are deciding whether or not to undertake screening for prostate cancer. Any reduction in prostate cancer-specific mortality may take up to 10 years to accrue; therefore, men who have a life expectancy less than 10 to 15 years should be informed that screening for prostate cancer is unlikely to be beneficial. No studies examined the independent role of screening by DRE.

Bottom Line: Screening with PSA only seems to help men less than 70

When to suspect prostate cancer

PSA by itself is a poor indicator and used as an excuse to do a biopsy. How fast PSA rises is more important and so is prostate size compared to PSA. A larger prostate with make more PSA.

PSA Velocity

According to two longitudinal studies, elevated PSA due to benign prostate enlargement should be stable or constantly rising with low velocity, <0.3 ng/ml/yr [1,2].

[1] Carter HB, Ferrucci L, Kettermann A, et al. Detection of life-threatening prostate cancer with prostate-specific antigen velocity during a window of curability. J Natl Cancer Inst 2006;98:1521–7.

[2] Berger AP, Deibl M, Strasak A, et al. Large-scale study of clinical impact of PSA velocity: long-term PSA kinetics as 640 european urology 52 (2007) 639–641 method of differentiating men with from those without prostate cancer. Urology 2007;69:34–8

J Natl Cancer Inst. 2006 Nov 1;98(21):1521-7.

Detection of life-threatening prostate cancer with prostate-specific antigen velocity during a window of curability.

RESULTS:

PSA velocity measured 10-15 years before diagnosis (when most men had PSA levels below 4.0 ng/mL) was associated with cancer-specific survival 25 years later; survival was

- 92% (95% confidence interval [CI] = 84% to 96%) among men with PSA velocity of 0.35 ng/mL per year or less
- 54% (95% CI = 15% to 82%) among men with PSA velocity above 0.35 ng/mL per year (P<.001).

PSA Density (PSAD)

PSA Density Higher Than 0.15 ng/cc Should Raise Concern about Prostate Cancer If a determination of the volume of the prostate has been made by ultrasound or some other radiological technique, we can calculate the PSA density (PSAD) or the amount of PSA (expressed in nanograms) for each cubic centimeter of the prostate volume. The PSAD is simply the serum PSA value divided by an accurate gland volume determination.

PSAD = Serum PSA ÷ Gland Volume (per TRUSP or Endorectal MRI)

Free PSA to Total PSA ratio

From: http://www.harvardprostateknowledge.org/

Whether you need both tests really depends on your individual situation. That's why this question generates so much debate and confusion.

PSA, a protein produced by prostate gland cells, circulates through the body in two ways: either bound to other proteins or on its own. PSA traveling alone is called free PSA. The free-PSA test measures the percentage of unbound PSA; the PSA test measures the total of both free and bound PSA.

Prostate cancer can raise PSA levels, but so can other conditions. These include an enlarged prostate, prostatitis, and advancing age. In fact, studies have shown that about 75% of men with an elevated PSA do not have prostate cancer. To determine which men actually have cancer and which don't, physicians traditionally perform a biopsy. Undergoing a biopsy isn't as traumatic as surgery, but it does cause discomfort and can provoke anxiety.

Rather than subject everyone with an elevated PSA to a biopsy, some urologists measure free PSA in patients with a total PSA level between 4 ng/ml and 10 ng/ml. Studies have shown that men with a total PSA in this "gray area" and a free PSA greater than 25% are more likely to have a benign condition than to have cancer, making a biopsy unnecessary. Men with a total PSA in the same range and a free PSA below 10% need to have a biopsy. More likely than not, they have prostate cancer (see table below).

In some cases, men with a "normal" PSA actually have cancer, but that low PSA doesn't prompt a biopsy. A low PSA and a low percentage of free PSA, however, probably would. That's why some doctors automatically order both tests at the same time. I tend to order a free-PSA test when a total PSA yields borderline results and when the PSA seems to be rising quickly, even if the actual number is relatively low. So, while the free-PSA test isn't essential, the results may sway your decision on whether to have a biopsy when combined with other tests. In the future, other tests may help determine whether changes in PSA are driven by cancerous tissue or benign causes.

Probability of finding prostate cancer based on % free PSA in men with a total PSA between 4 ng/ml and 10 ng/ml	
% free PSA	**Probability of prostate cancer**
0%–10%	56%
10%–15%	28%
15%–20%	20%
20%–25%	16%
Greater than 25%	8%
SOURCE: Journal of the American Medical Association, May 20, 1998.	

PSA Doubling Time

Japanese Journal of Clinical Oncology Volume 33, Issue 1Pp. 1-5

It was found that the PSA doubling time was a more powerful indicator of disease activity than standard histopathological criteria. We have started a non-randomized prospective observational study of watchful waiting for patients with T1c prostate cancer with favorable biopsy features, supported by the Ministry of Health, Labor and Welfare of Japan. In this multi-institutional study, we recommend watchful waiting for 6 months as an initial strategy for patients who fulfil the inclusion criteria shown in Table 1. After 6 months, we calculate the PSA doubling time based on four serial points (every 2 months) of PSA. If the patient shows a PSA doubling time of <2 years, we recommend aggressive treatment. For the rest of the patients, who show longer PSA doubling times, watchful waiting is recommended with PSA checking every 3 months and assessment of PSA doubling time every 6 months.

You can find a doubling time calculator here:

https://www.mskcc.org/nomograms/prostate/psa-doubling-time

PSA only

Once again, PSA testing alone can detect prostate cancer early, but testing 1,000 men every one to four years from age 55 to 69 has been shown to prevent up to one death from the disease. Also, PSA testing alone can lead to unneeded biopsies.

The latest research suggests that between 1 percent and 4 percent of men who have a prostate biopsy will develop an infection requiring **hospital** care. The 30-day hospital admission rate for infections increased from 0.6 percent in 1996 to 3.6 percent in 2005, according to a study of 75,190 Canadian men published in January 2013 in the Journal of Urology. A U.S. study of 17,472 men enrolled in Medicare covering a 16-year span found an increased rate of infections requiring hospitalization. The bump was seen toward the end of the study.

Men hospitalized with biopsy-related infections had a 12-fold higher risk of death compared to men who did not have a biopsy.

Survival rates for prostate cancer
According to the most recent data, when including *all* stages of prostate cancer:
- The 5-year relative survival rate is almost 100%
- The 10-year relative survival rate is 98%
- The 15-year relative survival rate is 95%

My Screening Recommendations

Based on hundreds of hours of research and personal experience

1. Get a baseline PSA at age 40 or younger if it is over 2 ng/ml get a Digital Rectal Exam (DRE)
2. Keep track of your PSA velocity if it is <0.3 ng/ml/yr. you are most likely in good shape.
3. If your PSA velocity is >0.3 ng/ml/yr. get a PSA density if it is 0.15 ng/ml. get an MRI or other radiation free imaging study.
4. If your PSA doubling time is less than 7 years get an MRI or other radiation free imaging study.
5. When I got my bad numbers and was scheduled for a biopsy I started my nutritional and supplements program and got my PSA back to normal in a few months. I cancelled my biopsy. As of this writing my PSAs have been lower than they were seven years ago. See chapter 36. MY PERSONAL JOURNEY.

4. BIOPSY

Cancer is almost always diagnosed by biopsy, a surgical procedure that removes tissue samples from tumors. The samples are viewed under a microscope by a pathologist to determine the presence and type of cancer. According to TMD Limited, a medical tourism company, it is the fear of biopsies spreading cancer that drives over half a million US citizens out of the country for medical treatment each year.

Doctors routinely recommend biopsies to diagnose cancer. PET and CT scans usually follow. PET uses a radioactive substance attached to sugar to find the cancer (cancer loves sugar). CT emits a powerful dose of radiation, in some cases equivalent to about 200 chest X-rays

All cells are surrounded by interstitial fluid. This fluid drains into the lymph system through lymph channels, to the upper left chest, where the major lymphatic channel drains directly into a blood vessel. When a scalpel or needle invades tissue with cancer cells, there will be some bleeding, spilling cancer cells into the blood vessels or the lymph system via the interstitial fluid. Once a few of the billions of cancer cells break away and enter the bloodstream, they travel to distant organs and start to grow. This process is called 'seeding'. The dangerously high amount of radiation in PET and CT scans damages normal cells, which produce abnormal cells when they divide, and those abnormal cells can become malignant.

When preforming prostate biopsies, doctors often aspirate cells from up to 30 different samples. Thirty chances for cancer to spread. While needle aspirations are safer than surgical biopsy, there are still dangers. According to Bloomberg News, patients having prostate needle biopsies are seeing an increasing number of anti-biotic resistant infections, such as E. coli. Two of every 100 men undergoing prostate biopsy will develop sepsis, a potentially lethal blood infection. Another study showed that 9 of 100,000 men who tested negative for cancer died within a month of their biopsy.

Breast biopsy complications can include pain, swelling, bleeding, and drainage from the biopsy site, infection and false positive results, leading to unnecessary treatments.

Doctors and researchers have noted that biopsy of a tumor can cause seeding, or spread of cancer cells along the path of the needle track at the biopsy site. Author and health researcher Karl Loren has documented 73 cases of seeding from biopsies causing metastasis on his website, KarlLoren.com.

Dr. Vincent Gammill, Center for the Study of Natural Oncology in Solana Beach, California, presented a case of a woman who had successfully treated her breast cancer naturally since 1994. Last year, her conventional oncologist convinced her that she was a fool to refuse a needle biopsy. She now has new tumors at each of the puncture sites.

"I rarely see distant metastasis until after a biopsy – and then it grows rapidly everywhere, especially in the bones," Gammill said.

In 2011, researchers for Mayo Clinic College of Medicine reported that transperitoneal biopsy of cancer of the bile duct is associated with a higher rate of peritoneal metastasis and they recommend the procedure not be performed if a curative method exists.

While conventional medical doctors must follow AMA protocol, many are questioning the wisdom of biopsies. And as patients become more educated, they are beginning to question the need for invasive and sometimes dangerous tests. There are tumor marker blood tests, ultrasounds, sonograms and MRIs that can also determine the presence of a tumor without risking the spread of cancer or infections. Patients who travel outside the country for safer testing and treatment are taking responsibility for their own healthcare.

Surprisingly, many alternative health centers outside the states still require biopsies. One small private clinic in Baja, Mexico does not. "Many patients come to us because they don't want to have a biopsy. Especially breast and prostate patients. We respect their wishes, and offer tumor marker testing, color Doppler sonograms, ultrasounds and whole body thermography instead," says Dr. Antonio Jimenez of Hope4Cancer Institute.

This clinic does not use any chemotherapy or radiation. They use a wide variety of mainstream treatments from around the world, including local and whole body hyperthermia, SonoPhoto Dynamic Therapy, immune modulation, IV therapy, natural vaccines, nutrition and detoxification among others. The treatments are painless, non-invasive and have no side effects.

Today patients are educated in a way that was not possible before the use of computers. Patients can do their own research and learn about the risks and side effects of treatments and procedures, and get a clear understanding of what is involved before they commit to treatment. The more patients learn, the better choices they can make. And because over half a million patients are going to Mexico and other countries for treatment, it appears that the choice is often to opt out of conventional modalities.

SOURCE TMD Limited

5. CT and PET Scans

CT emits a powerful dose of radiation, in some cases equivalent to about 200 chest X-rays, or the amount most people would be exposed to from natural sources over seven years.

According to some estimates, the radiation exposure a patient receives from a full-body CT scan is often 500 times that of a conventional X-ray and about the same as that received by people living 1.5 miles away from the center of the World War II atomic blasts in Japan.

That dose can alter the makeup of human tissue and create free radicals, molecules that can wreak havoc on human cells. Your body can often repair that damage— but not always. And when it doesn't, the damage can lead to cancer.

Cancers from medical radiation can take anywhere from five to 60 years to develop, and risk also depends on age and lifestyle. That's why scientists struggled in early attempts to quantify the danger of medical radiation. Until recently, researchers often relied on evidence from the atomic bomb attacks on Hiroshima and Nagasaki. But now research shows that today's medical patients are being harmed, too.

New evidence comes from a 2013 Australian study that looked at more than 680,000 people who had CT scans as children and compared them with some 10 million children who did not have a CT scan. The researchers determined that for every 10,000 young people scanned, 45 would develop cancer over the next 10 years, compared with 39 cancers among 10,000 people not screened. Overall, people scanned had a 24 percent increased cancer risk, and each additional scan boosted risk an additional 16 percent. Children who had one before the age of 5 faced a 35 percent spike in cancer risk, reflecting the fact that young bodies are more vulnerable to radiation.

Positron Emission Tomography (PET) scans

PET scans differ from other types of diagnostic imaging in that they allow doctors to see how an organ or system is *functioning* rather than just seeing the *structure*. This test works in a very different way than other tests and does not use x-rays-rather, it uses gamma rays, which usually have a higher level of energy than x-rays.

PET scans work by injecting (or swallowing) small amounts of radioactive material, which then spreads throughout the body. The PET scanner is then used to detect the radiation that is emitting from the radioactive material in your body. Procedures that use radioactive material to diagnose and treat patients is referred to as "nuclear medicine."

The dose of radiation from a PET scan is similar to CT, and therefore exposes people to a relatively high dose of radiation in comparison to other types of scans.

6. TREATMENT (TRADITIONAL MEDICINE)

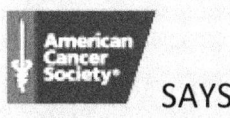 SAYS:

COMPARING WATCHFUL WAITING OR ACTIVE SURVEILLANCE WITH ACTIVE TREATMENT

A few large studies have compared **watchful waiting** (where men were treated only if they developed symptoms from their cancer) and surgery for early stage prostate cancer, but the evidence from these studies has been mixed. Some have found that men who have surgery might live longer, while others have not found a difference in survival.

So far, no large studies have compared **active surveillance** to treatments such as surgery or radiation therapy. Some early studies of men who are good candidates for active surveillance have shown that only about a third of the men need to go on to treatment with radiation or surgery.

Last Medical Review: 02/16/2016
Last Revised: 03/11/2016

WebMD News from HealthDay

By Randy Dotinga

HealthDay Reporter

TUESDAY, July 7, 2015 (HealthDay News) -- More U.S. physicians are sparing their low-risk prostate cancer patients from surgery, radiation and hormone therapy in favor of monitoring their patients over time -- a strategy called watchful waiting, a new study shows.

The number of low-risk patients who didn't undergo treatment jumped from as low as 7 percent from 1990-2009 to 40 percent from 2010-2013, the study revealed. These findings indicate that more patients are being monitored to see if their conditions get worse.

This is "excellent news" about the popularity of "active surveillance," said study author Dr. Matthew Cooperberg, the Helen Diller Family Chair in Urology at the University of California, San Francisco.

"We expected to see a rise in surveillance rates, but were surprised by the steepness of the trajectory," he said. "This really does represent a paradigm change, and it's faster than the typical pace of medical evolution."

The reason for the debate over who gets treated is that prostate cancer treatments, such as surgery or radiation, can lead to serious long-term side effects, such as incontinence and impotence. In addition, some prostate cancers are slow-growing and are less likely to cause problems, especially for older men, the American Cancer Society notes.

Last week, a study in the journal *JAMA Internal Medicine* suggested that the wide majority of men with low-risk prostate cancer between 2010 and 2011 had treatment. But, that study defined low-risk in various ways that included between 11 percent and 40 percent of prostate cancer patients.

The new study examines the medical records of more than 10,000 men from 45 urology practices. And, it uses a single definition of low-risk. The current study also looks at information through 2013.

In addition to finding a higher rate of watchful waiting in all men, the study also found that those aged 75 and older were much less likely to get potentially unnecessary treatment. Among low-risk men aged 75 and older, the rate of watchful waiting shot up from 22 percent in 2000-2004 to 76 percent in 2010-2013, the study found.

As for patients at greater danger, "we're seeing more aggressive management of higher- risk disease with surgery, radiation or both, which is also a trend toward better management," Cooperberg said.

But, the findings aren't necessarily all positive.

"Ultimately, the number of men who will die of prostate cancer because they chose active surveillance cannot be zero by definition," Cooperberg acknowledged. "But it is a very low number, far lower by most estimations than the number of those harmed by avoidable surgery, radiation, etc."

Dr. David Penson, the Hamilton and Howd Chair in Urologic Oncology at Vanderbilt University Medical Center in Nashville, Tenn., agreed with Cooperberg that the statistics are "very good news."

"The net health benefit for men with prostate cancer is likely more positive because we are treating the men who need treatment while we are avoiding the risk of side effects in those who don't," he said.

Also, he said, the findings have implications for the debate about screening men for prostate cancer via "PSA" blood tests.

"One of the arguments against screening is that we are over-detecting and overtreating prostate cancer, and because we are overtreating men who don't need treatment, we are doing more harm than good. By reducing the rates of overtreatment, we are likely increasing the benefit of screening," he noted.

The study appears in the July 7 2015, issue of *Journal of the American Medical Association*.

Radical prostatectomy (surgery). The surgeon removes the prostate and seminal vesicles (saclike glands that release fluid that becomes part of semen). In some cases, pelvic lymph nodes are also sampled. This is most often performed through an abdominal incision; abdominal surgery may also be done with a laparoscope. A third option is the perineal technique, involving an incision in the area between the scrotum and the anus (the perineum). The most common side effects are

- impotence (affecting 30%–70% of men)

- mild to severe incontinence (2%–15%).

Men with no evidence of prostate cancer spread have an 85% chance of surviving 10 years after radical prostatectomy.

External beam radiation therapy. After a CT scan constructs a three-dimensional picture of the prostate and seminal vesicles, the radiation oncologist directs rays of high-energy radiation at the prostate tumor and sometimes at nearby lymph nodes. The most common side effects are

- impotence (30%–70%)
- mild to severe incontinence (1%–2%).

Brachytherapy. With ultrasound guidance, radioactive "seeds" or pellets are implanted in the prostate itself to irradiate the tumor. The most common side effects are

- impotence (30%–50%)
- mild to severe incontinence (2%).

Active surveillance. This involves an extended period of monitoring the cancer with regular digital rectal exams, PSA tests, and sometimes repeated prostate biopsies. If tests indicate cancer has become active, treatment options are offered. The major risk of active surveillance is that the cancer could become active during the period of surveillance, potentially making prognosis worse.

There are more side effects than were reported to their doctor

Most patients don't always talk openly with their doctors about the impact treatment has had on their quality of life or doctors don't ask.

Fecal incontinence. A telephone survey of 227 men with prostate cancer revealed that 5% of those who underwent radical prostatectomy and 18% of those who had a perineal prostatectomy developed fecal incontinence afterward. Yet fewer than 50% told their physicians. (Source: Bishoff JT, Motley G, Optenberg SA, et al. Incidence of Fecal and Urinary Incontinence Following Radical Perineal and Retropubic Prostatectomy in a National Population. *Journal of Urology* 1998;160:454–8. PMID: 9679897.)

Erectile dysfunction. A mailed questionnaire returned by 1,236 men with localized prostate cancer who had undergone either prostatectomy or radiation therapy revealed that 36% had erectile dysfunction at the time of diagnosis. Yet when contacted an average of four years after treatment, more than twice as many men (85%) said they had erectile dysfunction. Only 13% were able to have firm, reliable erections spontaneously. Respondents indicated that they were as concerned about the loss of sexual desire and the ability to have an orgasm as they were about erectile dysfunction. (Source: Schover LR, Fouladi RT, Warneke CL, et al.

Defining Sexual Outcomes after Treatment for Localized Prostate Carcinoma. *Cancer* 2002;95:1773–85. PMID: 12365027.)

Urinary incontinence. A retrospective analysis based on Medicare claims submitted by 11,522 men who underwent prostatectomy for prostate cancer found that more than one year after surgery, 18%–24% (the proportion increased with age) had suffered symptoms of urinary incontinence or had undergone procedures to correct urinary difficulties. (Source: Begg CB, Riedel ER, Bach PB, et al. Variations in Morbidity after Radical Prostatectomy. *New England Journal of Medicine* 2002;346:1138–44. PMID: 11948274.)

Rectal cancer risk. A retrospective analysis of the outcomes of 30,552 men who received radiation for prostate cancer found that they were almost twice as likely to develop rectal cancer as a comparison group of 55,263 men who treated their cancer with surgery. (Source: Baxter NN, Tepper JE, Durham SB, et al. Increased Risk of Rectal Cancer after Prostate Radiation: A Population-Based Study. *Gastroenterology* 2005;128:819–24. PMID: 15825064.)

Prostate Cancer Vaccine

This vaccine is designed to treat, not prevent, prostate cancer by spurring your body's immune system to attack prostate cancer cells. Immune cells are removed from your blood, activated to fight cancer, and infused back into the blood. Three cycles occur in one month. It's used for advanced prostate cancer that no longer responds to hormone therapy. Mild side effects can occur such as fatigue, nausea, and fever.

There are a number of trials for several types of prostate cancer vaccines. So far they haven't cured only extended life 4 to 7 months. For updates go to:

http://www.cancerresearch.org/prostate-cancer

Nutritional Treatment

7. Flaxseed

Much of the following information on nutrients was based on: Life Extension Magazine December 2013 A Natural Arsenal for Prostate Cancer Prevention By Michael Downey

Studies have shown that flaxseed supplementation lowers PSA levels, and significantly reduces the proliferation of normal prostate cells and prostate cancer cells.

Dr. OZ recommends flaxseed lignans on his website. Here is a quote from www.doctoroz.com, "Flax contains lignans which reduce the risk of breast cancer in women and prostate cancer in men. The lignans alter the way your body metabolizes estrogens into safer forms."

From http://www.lifescript.com

Lignans are naturally occurring chemicals widespread within the plant and animal kingdoms. Several lignans— with intimidating names such as secoisolariciresinol— are considered to be phytoestrogens, plant chemicals that mimic the hormone estrogen. These are especially abundant in flaxseeds and sesame seeds. Bacteria in our intestines convert the naturally occurring phytoestrogens from flaxseed into two other lignans, enterolactone and enterodiol, which also have estrogen-like effects. In this article, the term lignans refers to these two specific lignans as well as the phytoestrogen kind, but not to the wide variety of other lignans.

Lignans are being studied for possible use in cancer prevention, particularly breast cancer. Like other phytoestrogens (such as soy isoflavones), they hook onto the same spots on cells where estrogen attaches. If there is little estrogen in the body (after menopause, for example), lignans may act like weak estrogen; but when natural estrogen is abundant in the body, lignans may instead reduce estrogen's effects by displacing it from cells. This displacement of the hormone may help prevent those cancers, such as breast cancer, that depend on estrogen to start and develop. In addition, at least one test tube study suggests that lignans may help prevent cancer in ways that are unrelated to estrogen. 1

Requirements/Sources

The richest source of lignans is flaxseed (sometimes called linseed), containing more than 100 times the amount found in other foods! Flaxseed oil , however, does not contain appreciable amounts of lignans. Sesame seed is an equally rich source. Other food sources are pumpkin seeds, whole grains, cranberries, and black or green tea.

Therapeutic Dosages

The University of Maryland Medical Center recommends adults consume 1 tablespoon of ground flaxseed two to three times a day, or 2 to 4 tablespoons once per day. You can mix the ground seeds into cereal, yogurt, oatmeal or smoothies or sprinkle them generously on top of salads and vegetable dishes.

Enterolactones from flax protect against hormone-dependent cancers. Tyrosine kinases are activated in metastatic prostate cancer cells, and enterolactones help to inhibit the tyrosine kinase enzyme. Enterolactones have been shown to inhibit *5-alpha-reductase*, an enzyme that converts testosterone to a more potent androgen. Anti-angiogenesis effects and cancer-cell apoptosis were found to be enhanced by enterolactones in animal models of hormone-related cancers, including prostate cancer. Enterolactone also functions via several mechanisms to reduce estrogen input to cells and has been shown in a number of studies to be a factor in the development of benign prostate enlargement and prostate cancer.

Researchers had men who were about to get their prostates removed eat 3 tablespoons of flaxseeds a day for the few weeks before surgery. They were skeptical that they would observe any differences in tumor biology between the flaxseed-fortified diet-treated patients and the controls with such a short-term dietary intervention, but they found significantly lower cancer proliferation rates and significantly higher rates of apoptotic cell death, the cancer cell suicide.

Mammalian lignan precursors as aglycones (μg / 100 g). Major compound(s) in bold.

Foodstuff	Pinoresinol	Syringaresinol	Sesamin	Lariciresinol
Flaxseed	871	48	not detected	1780
Sesame seed	**47136**	205	**62724**	13060
Rye bran	**1547**	**3540**	nd	**1503**
Wheat bran	138	882	nd	672
Oat bran	**567**	297	nd	**766**
Barley bran	71	140	nd	133

Foodstuff	Secoisolariciresinol	Matairesinol	Hydroxymatairesinol
Flaxseed	**165759**	529	35
Sesame seed	240	1137	7209
Rye bran	**1503**	729	1017
Wheat bran	672	410	**2787**
Oat bran	**766**	440	**712**
Barley bran	133	42	**541**

nd not detected

8. BORON

Life Extension Magazine November 2015
Boron Reduces Prostate Cancer Risk
By Michael Downey

Boron has been found to selectively kill prostate cancer cells while leaving healthy cells unharmed. In addition, boron has been found to lower PSA—which was previously believed to be only a marker for prostate cancer. More recent research shows that elevated PSA is a causative factor in prostate cancer progression.

Adequate boron levels are associated with a 64% reduced risk of prostate cancer, but obtaining protective levels of boron from food alone is difficult. This means that supplementation with low-cost boron could be a lifesaver for aging males at risk for prostate cancer, in addition to other health benefits provided by this vital mineral.

The idea that supplemental use of boron might reduce the risk of prostate cancer was first brought to the attention of scientists following a 2001 study on dietary patterns of prostate cancer patients as reported long ago in Life Extension magazine.

This study compared the diets of 76 prostate cancer patients with those of 7,651 men without cancer. Researchers found that men who ingested the greatest amount of boron from their diets were 64% less likely to develop prostate cancer than those who consumed the least.

Interestingly, while there was a significant decrease in cancer risk in the group that consumed the most boron, those in the highest intake group only consumed 2.5 additional servings of fruit and one additional serving of nuts per day compared to those in the lowest boron intake group.

A subsequent study confirmed these findings. For the study, the researchers compared the dietary boron intake of 95 prostate cancer patients with that of 8,720 healthy male controls. Researchers controlled for age, race, education, smoking, body mass index, dietary caloric intake, and alcohol consumption. They found that men with the highest boron intake showed a 54% lower risk of prostate cancer compared to those with the lowest intake. In addition, they noted that increased dietary boron intake was associated with a decreased risk of prostate cancer in a dose-response manner.

These findings not only underscored the remarkable, broad-spectrum health benefits associated with consuming fruits, but also suggested that boron in particular may be responsible for some of these protective benefits.

Encouraged by these epidemiological findings showing a connection between dietary intake of boron and reduced risk for prostate cancer, scientists set out to determine if supplementing with boron could protect against prostate cancer. Initial animal studies indicate that the answer is yes.

In a validated animal model of prostate cancer, researchers found that oral administration of various concentrations of a boron-containing solution substantially decreased tumor size. It also lowered levels of prostate-specific antigen or PSA—the most abundant protein synthesized in the prostate gland—suggesting a possible mechanism for these anticancer effects.

In this animal model, researchers orally administered various concentrations of a boron-containing solution to test subjects and found that this resulted in decreases in prostate tumor size by 25% to 38%. Remarkably, PSA levels dropped by an astounding 86% to 89% in the animals that received boron.

These findings suggested that supplemental boron may have both preventive and therapeutic effects—helping both to shrink prostate tumors and to decrease levels of PSA.

Novel Protective Mechanisms

The finding that supplemental boron can help to shrink prostate tumors while also decreasing levels of PSA7 is particularly exciting. At one time, PSA was viewed primarily as a blood indicator of prostate cancer, infection, or inflammation. However, evidence now reveals that PSA plays a critical role in the progression and metastasis of prostate cancer, thus opening up new therapeutic pathways for preventing and treating this epidemic disease with PSA-lowering nutrients such as boron.

Scientists now believe that elevated PSA breaks down the protein surrounding the cells (called the extra-cellular protein matrix) within the prostate gland. The breakdown of these cellular barriers by excess PSA may be what enables prostate cancer cells to more readily invade healthy tissue and spread themselves beyond the prostate gland, with potentially lethal consequences. This remarkable data provides further understanding as to how we may prevent or slow down prostate cancer by reducing PSA levels.

Published evidence further suggests that higher intake of boron-containing compounds can inhibit PSA activity and lower the risk of prostate cancer by reducing intracellular calcium signals and storage.

Boron is increasingly recognized for its targeted capacity to destroy prostate cancer cells and lower prostate-specific antigen, or PSA—while leaving healthy cells unharmed.

Boron quantities found in food are usually very low.

Adequate boron intake via supplements may help prevent or control potentially lethal prostate cancer and support optimum health.

Using Boron As Adjuvant Treatment

A number of studies have led researchers to conclude that boron could have specific therapeutic potential in the treatment of prostate cancer.

Less well-known than PSA is a protein called prostate specific membrane antigen or PSMA. While PSMA has not yet been completely verified as a marker for prostate cancer, studies have shown that the expression of PSMA in tumors and metastases of men with prostate cancer is greater than PSMA in men without prostate cancer.

In 2014, scientists published a cell study based on the ability of boron to inhibit PSMA. They found that boron-rich compounds demonstrated significant uptake by prostate cancer cells, which indicated that boron compounds may be useful in developing a new class of therapeutic agents—among those known as boron neutron capture therapy or BCNT—against prostate cancer. BCNT is a type of noninvasive, injection-based anticancer therapy using boron.

Another aspect of boron that makes it an especially beneficial therapeutic agent is its ability to selectively inhibit the growth of prostate cancer cells while still allowing normal prostate cells to grow. Scientists know that these actions are dose-dependent, though the underlying mechanism for this targeted effect is still under investigation.

A 2014 study published in Tumour Biology, however, did reveal that a compound containing boron induced apoptosis, or cell death, in prostate cancer cells. The researchers were able to determine that the boron agent disrupted the normal organization of prostate cancer cells' actin filaments, which are threadlike, protein fibers that are an essential element or building block of the cell. The compound containing boron exerted other cytotoxic or cell-killing effects, including the reduction of telomerase activity in the cancer cells.

They concluded that the boron in this compound "could be an important agent for its therapeutic potential in the treatment of prostate cancer."

The increasingly evident conclusion is that ensuring an adequate daily boron intake via supplementation—and not relying on the small and extremely variable amounts of boron available in plant foods from different agricultural regions—represents an important component of a strategy to prevent prostate cancer and maintain optimal PSA levels.

In fact, emerging studies now suggest that boron delivers another layer of protection against the symptoms of this prostate cancer—in the bone.

The major and most deadly danger in prostate cancer is its ability to spread to the bone, which is its natural evolution. Bone is the initial and main site for about 80% of all prostate cancer metastases. They occur most commonly in the spine, pelvis, ribs, skull, and proximal femur.

These bone metastases induce significant skeletal remodeling, fractures, anemia, and pain—and are a major cause of morbidity and mortality. Prostate cancer has been described as "uniformly lethal once it has escaped the confines of the prostate gland." Sadly, the median survival of patients after prostate cancer has spread to the bone is 40 months.

Although more studies are needed, boron's remarkably targeted capacity to inhibit the spread of prostate cancer cells while sparing normal cells may have the same targeted effect against prostate cancer cells that have migrated to the bone. With wider boron supplementation, this cytotoxic effect—combined with boron's potential to help prevent prostate cancer from occurring in the first place—could reduce the current 28,000 American deaths from this disease every year.

Boron is a trace mineral that is essential to plant growth and finds its way into the human diet through our consumption of plant foods—especially apples, plums, grapes, avocados, vegetables, nuts, and legumes.

Despite its widespread availability in plant foods, ingesting adequate amounts of boron through dietary choices can be difficult. Why? Because the total quantity of boron in any one plant food is very low.

For example, apples are considered to be a good source of boron. However, to attain the minimum 3 mg daily intake of boron that is generally suggested, you would need to eat about 2.4 pounds of apples a day—that's over eight apples! You wouldn't have to worry about surpassing the tolerable daily intake (TDI) for boron until you managed to consume about 68 apples during a single day!

Worse, with modern dietary habits, many individuals can develop a boron deficiency by simply failing to eat enough fruits, vegetables, and nuts. And even among those whose diets include rich quantities of these plant foods, their boron intake will be greatly affected by regional geology because the food content of boron varies greatly according to the boron content of the soil in the region where the produce was grown. Even local preferences for some foods over others can result in high or low human boron levels.

Ensuring optimal boron intake becomes increasingly important as we age. While boron has long been recognized for its critical role in safeguarding bone health, scientists are increasingly excited about growing evidence of boron's powerful role in blocking the development of prostate cancer.

9. CRUCIFEROUS VEGETABLES

Cruciferous vegetables (broccoli, Brussels sprouts, cabbage, collards, cauliflower, kale, mustard greens, turnips, and rutabagas, watercress) have four important cancer fighting compounds: **Indole-3-carbinol (IC3), Diindolymethane (DIM), Phenethyl Isothiocyanate (PEITC) and apigenin.**

Indole-3-carbinol (I3C) has several different actions that help prevent and inhibit prostate cancer. It helps activate detoxification pathways, prevents cancer cell growth, induces apoptosis, regulates gene expression, protects DNA from damage, and modulates a variety of cell signaling pathways.

WebMD says:

Indole-3-carbinol is used for prevention of breast cancer, colon cancer, and other types of cancer. The National Institutes of Health (NIH) has reviewed indole-3-carbinol as a possible cancer preventive agent and is now sponsoring clinical research for breast cancer prevention.

Indole-3-carbinol is also used for fibromyalgia, tumors inside the voice box (laryngeal papillomatosis) caused by a virus, tumors inside the respiratory tract (respiratory papillomatosis) caused by a virus, abnormal cell growth in the cervix (cervical dysplasia), and systemic lupus erythematosus (SLE). Some people use indole-3-carbinol to balance hormone levels, "detoxify" the intestines and liver, and to support the immune system.

Diindolymethane (DIM) has been shown to protect against prostate cancer by inhibiting the phosphorus-transferring enzyme **Akt**, inhibiting the master DNA-transcription regulator **nuclear factor-kappaB (NF-kB)**— and blocking the crosstalk between them. This is a novel mechanism through which DIM inhibits cell growth and induces apoptosis in prostate cancer cells, but not in non-tumorigenic prostate epithelial cells.

In a study released in May 2013, PEITC was found to suppress a compound known as **PROSTATE CANCER (P300/CBP-associated factor)**—which in turn inhibits androgen receptor-regulated transcriptional activity in prostate cancer cells.

In studies on human cancer cells, scientists observed that the vegetable extract apigenin inhibits angiogenesis and cell proliferation. These effects were confirmed in an animal experiment in which scientists transplanted an androgen-dependent line of human prostate cancer cells into mice bred to serve as a model for tumor growth conditions. A liquid suspension containing either apigenin or placebo was given to the mice daily, via a gastric tube, for eight or ten weeks. Administering apigenin to mice—beginning either two weeks before, or two weeks after, inoculation with the cells—inhibited the volume of prostate cancer cells in a dose-dependent manner by as much as **59%** and **53%**, respectively. Induction of apoptosis in the tumor xenografts was observed. In the same study, exposure of prostate cancer cells to apigenin in a culture for as little as 24 hours appeared to inhibit cell cycle progression by nearly **69%**.

Scientists believe these effects may result from apigenin's modulation of the IGF (***insulin-like growth factors***) axis, which plays signaling roles in cell proliferation and cell death. Later research demonstrated that apigenin also inhibits motility and invasiveness of prostate carcinoma cells.

10. VITAMIN D

In recent years, a multitude of studies have shown cancer risk reductions of **50%** and greater based on higher vitamin D status. People with higher vitamin D levels have lower risks of lethal prostate cancer, as well as reduced risks of other cancers. In 2011, Dr. Garland's team found that a vitamin D level of 50 ng/ml is associated with a 50 percent lower risk of breast cancer (Similarly, a 2007 study published in the *American Journal of Preventive Medicine* concluded that a vitamin D level of more than 33 ng/mL was associated with a 50 percent lower risk of colorectal cancer.)

To reach a minimum protective level of 40 ng/ml of vitamin D, study participants had to take anywhere from 1,000 IUs to as much as 8,000 IUs of vitamin D3 per day—a far cry from the recommended daily allowance of 600 IUs of vitamin D for adults.

The supplemental dose ensuring that 97.5 percent of the study population achieved a serum 25(OH)D of at least 40 ng/mL was 9,600 IU/day. This study also concluded that intake of up to 40,000 IUs per day is unlikely to result in vitamin D toxicity.

While numerous studies show people with higher blood levels of vitamin D have lowered cancer risk, what had been lacking was a double blind, placebo-controlled study that specifically measured the effects of higher-dose vitamin D supplementation (with calcium) on cancer incidence in humans. This is the kind of study that conventional medical doctors insist on seeing if they are to believe a nutrient (or drug) really provides a health benefit.

In a breakthrough report, the effects of administering 1,000 IU a day of vitamin D (with calcium) was evaluated in 1,180 postmenopausal women living in the Midwest.10

After four years, the risk of contracting any cancer was **60% lower** in the vitamin D (and calcium) group, compared with the placebo arm of the study.

The scientists then performed an even more detailed analysis of the data. When excluding cancers diagnosed in the first year of the study, which would have included preexisting cancers present at the time participants began taking vitamin D, they found an astounding **77% reduction** in cancer incidence in the group receiving vitamin D, compared with placebo. (Interestingly, in a third arm of this study in which the participants received calcium but no vitamin D, the cancer risk reductions were not as significant.)

What this means is that if all Americans began taking just 1,000 IU of vitamin D each day (with calcium), as many as three-quarters of all cancers could be prevented in just four years.

11. Soy Isoflavones

Japanese scientists took blood samples from over 14,000 men during 1988-1990. Their analysis clearly established that elevated serum levels of all three isoflavones assessed—*genistein*, *daidzein*, and *equol*—imparted strong protective effects against prostate cancer. Men with the highest circulating levels of genistein, daidzein, and equol reduced prostate cancer risk by **62%**, **59%**, and **66%**, respectively. Genistein and daidzein are found in soy, and equol is derived from daidzein by bacterial flora in the intestines. Also, genistein was shown to have "potent anti-proliferative effects" against human prostate cells and inhibit metastatic potential of sex gland cancers such as prostate cancer. Genistein also blocks an enzyme that destroys an anticancer vitamin D metabolite in cancer cells.

12. GREEN TEA EXTRACT

A clinical trial demonstrated that green tea catechins were **90%** effective in preventing prostate cancer in men with pre-malignant lesions. Researchers recruited 60 men, aged 45-75. Thirty participants received **200 milligrams** of green tea catechins (**50%** EGCG) **three times daily**, while the other 30 subjects received a placebo. Biopsies were conducted at six and 12 months. Remarkably, only **one** man in the treatment group was diagnosed with prostate cancer, compared to **nine** men in the control group who developed the disease. No significant side effects or adverse reactions were reported. The lead researcher concluded that "**90%** of chemoprevention efficacy could be obtained by [green tea catechin] administration in men prone to developing prostate cancer".

Green tea polyphenols have also shown efficacy as an adjunctive therapy. Prostate cancer patients were given **1,300 milligrams** of green tea polyphenols, mostly EGCG, prior to the time of radical prostatectomy. They showed significant reductions in PSA and other tumor promoters such as *vascular endothelial growth factor*.

13. OMEGA-3 FATTY ACIDS

EPA has been shown to suppress the formation of the omega-6 fatty acid **arachidonic acid** (AA) by inhibiting the enzyme **delta-5-desaturase**. EPA has also been found to contribute to the inhibition of **uPA** —a substance known as **urokinase-type plasminogen activator** believed to play a role in prostate cancer invasion and metastasis.

14. Curcumin

Both *in vitro* and *in vivo* models demonstrate that curcumin inhibits prostate cancer promotion by blocking metastases of cancer cells in the prostate, and by regulating enzymes required for tissue invasiveness. In certain human prostate cancer cell lines, curcumin completely inhibited a type of phosphorus-transferring enzyme known as **Akt** (also known as **protein kinase B** or **PKB**), suggesting that curcumin inhibits prostate cancer cell growth through this Akt-inhibiting mechanism. Curcumin has been shown to inhibit angiogenesis in prostate cancer cells *in vivo*.

15. COENZYME Q10

University of Miami researchers reported research showing that adding coenzyme Q10 *in vitro* to the most common prostate cancer cell line, PC3, inhibited cell growth by **70%** over 48 hours. Evidence suggested that there had been a reduction in the expression of a key, anti-apoptotic gene protein, bcl-2, and through this mechanism, CoQ10 had restored the ability for apoptosis, allowing the cancer cells to kill themselves. "The most amazing part," said UM research associate Niven Narain, "is that we've been able to restore a cancer cell's ability to kill itself, while not impacting normal cells."

16. GAMMA-TOCOPHEROL VITAMIN E

A large study showed that the risk of prostate cancer declines with increasing concentrations of the **alpha**-tocopherol form of vitamin E, with the highest level corresponding to a **35% lower** risk; however, these protective effects were **only** observed when levels of **gamma**-tocopherol and levels of selenium were also high.

17. LYCOPENE

Lycopene is a carotenoid occurring abundantly in tomatoes. The relationship between its ingestion and prostate health is well established. One laboratory experiment found that lycopene inhibited the growth of normal human prostate cells. Then, a clinical trial conducted on prostate cancer patients demonstrated that lycopene supplementation decreases the growth of prostate cancer. In another compelling study, healthy men with the highest lycopene levels in their blood were shown to have a **60%** reduced risk of developing prostate cancer. Three studies have examined serum carotenoids using prediagnostic samples in relation to prostate cancer risk. The first study, which was based on serum obtained in 1974 from 25 802 persons in Washington County, MD, found a 6.2% lower median lycopene level in prostate cancer case subjects diagnosed during 13 years compared with age- and race-matched control subjects. The estimated RR was 0.50 (95% CI = 0.20-1.29) between high and low quartiles of lycopene. No other carotenoid was associated with prostate cancer risk. Preliminary results from the Physicians' Health Study, which was based on 581 case subjects, found a statistically significant RR of 0.56 (95% CI = 0.34-0.91) when comparing high quintile with low quintile of plasma lycopene.

Scientists found that lycopene works by reducing oxidative stress in prostate tissue; lowering inflammatory signaling; preventing DNA damage; modulating expression of endocrine growth factors; and may block cancer cells from growing out of control through enhanced communication between cancer cells at "gap junctions". Lycopene also may slow the new blood vessel growth that prostate cancers need for development.

18. ZINC

Evidence suggests that zinc may play an important and direct role in the prostate. For example, studies found that total zinc levels in the prostate are much higher than in other soft tissues in the body, and those with prostate cancer have been shown to have exceedingly low levels of zinc in the prostate. Also, in normal prostate cells, zinc is highly concentrated intracellularly in the glandular epithelium—but adenocarcinoma cells taken from prostate tumors have lost their ability to amass zinc. Supplementation with **15 milligrams of zinc daily** showed a trend toward modestly reduced risk of all invasive prostate cancers, but there was a significant **66%** reduction in risk of advanced prostate cancer. This indicates that zinc supplements may be beneficial in some subgroups of men for the most advanced forms of the disease. There was also a greater reduction in prostate cancer risk from zinc supplementation among men whose vegetable intake was high.

19. Milk Thistle

In animal research, silibinin was found to exert cancer-fighting effects against an advanced form of human prostate tumor cells, resulting in decreased proliferation and increased cancer-cell apoptosis. Silibinin has high bioavailability in the prostate after oral administration, and scientists concluded that it has strong potential to be developed as an intervention for hormone-refractory (castration-resistant) human prostate cancer. Silibinin may also work synergistically with the chemotherapy drug **doxorubicin** to help kill cancer cells, making it a potential candidate for adjuvant therapy.

20. GAMMA-LINOLENIC ACID (GLA)

GLA has been found to inhibit the production of **urokinase-type plasminogen activator (uPA)**, a substance believed to play a role in the invasiveness and metastasis of cancer cells.

Scientists have also found that GLA metabolites suppress the activity of **5alpha-reductase**, an enzyme that converts testosterone to a more potent androgen (**5alpha-dihydrotestosterone or DHT**) and that is involved in the pathway of prostate cancer. It is believed that GLA may also increase the effectiveness of some anticancer drug treatments.

21. ZEAXANTHIN

In a 2001 study, a scientific team analyzed the plasma levels of various substances in a group of participants that included 65 patients with prostate cancer and 132 cancer-free controls. They found that, relative to those in the lowest quartile, those in the highest quartile of plasma zeaxanthin had a **78%** reduced risk of prostate cancer.

22. POMEGRANATE

Use of pomegranate (*Punica granatum* L. var. *spinosa*) juice, peel, and oil has been shown to possess anticancer activities, including interference with tumor cell proliferation, cell cycle, invasiveness, and angiogenesis. Apoptosis was implicated as a mechanism for this interference with prostate cancer cell proliferation in a laboratory study in which researchers found that pomegranate extract increases expression of a protein that promotes cancer cell death, while decreasing expression of a protein that inhibits cancer cell death. Later, in a 2012 study, scientists found that the in vitro cytotoxic activity of an extract of pomegranate against prostate cancer cells was dose-dependent—and they also suggested that this antiproliferative effect followed an apoptosis-dependent pathway.

Further clarifying pomegranate's effects against prostate cancer cells, scientists found evidence of induced beneficial gene expression—inhibiting pro-inflammatory, DNA-related protein **nuclear factor kappa B (NF-kB)** and downregulating production of cancer-stimulating androgen receptors in prostate cells.

According to a study presented at the American Urological Association's annual meeting in 2009, drinking 8 ounces of pomegranate juice a day may slow the progression of prostate cancer.

The study included 48 men who had a rising prostate-specific antigen (PSA) level following radiation therapy or surgery to treat localized prostate cancer. At the start of the study in 2003, the men had PSA levels greater than 0.2 and less than 5.0 ng/ml, and an average PSA doubling time of 15.4 months. (PSA doubling time is a measure of cancer's activity, with shorter times indicating more aggressive behavior.) In 2006, researchers reported that the men who drank 8 ounces of pomegranate juice daily had slower PSA doubling times.

Since then, researchers continued to follow the participants, 15 of whom stuck with the study for as long as 64 months. They found that the PSA doubling times of the men who kept drinking pomegranate juice were about four times longer than the PSA doubling times at the study's start — and longer than the PSA doubling times of the men who stopped drinking the juice.

For those who want to try pomegranate juice, one note of caution: it's high in calories. An 8-ounce glass of POM Wonderful, the juice used in the study, contains 160 calories, 50 calories more than a typical glass of orange juice.

SOURCE: Pantuck AJ, Zomorodian N, Rettig M, et al. Long-term Follow-Up of Phase 2 Study of Pomegranate Juice for Men with Prostate Cancer Shows Durable Prolongation of PSA Doubling Time. Journal of Urology 2009;181(4 Suppl): abstract 826.

23. SAW PALMETTO

Saw palmetto extract to slow the growth of prostate cancer cells *in vitro*. This growth-inhibitory effect was **more potent** on prostate cancer cells than on other cancer cell lines on which they tested saw palmetto. One new mechanism identified by this group of scientists was the saw palmetto-induced reduction in the expression of *cyclooxygenase-2 (COX-2)* in prostate cancer cells. Cancer cells often use COX-2 as biological fuel to hyper-proliferate, and as the researchers presenting this report concluded, "We hypothesize that COX-2 inhibition induced by saw palmetto berry extract may provide an important basis for potential chemopreventative action."

24. RESVERATROL

By working through over a dozen anticancer mechanisms and selectively targeting cancer cells, resveratrol inhibits prostate cancer at multiple stages of development. This potent compound, found in grapes and other plants, was first isolated in 1940 and is now viewed as a potential defense against this disease. In a study that examined the effect of various polyphenols on different types of prostate cancer cells, scientists concluded that resveratrol was the most potent against advanced prostate cancer cells.

Resveratrol has the ability to modulate the activity of estrogen and testosterone at both the cellular (receptor) and molecular (genetic) levels. In fact, after examining its effects on hormone-responsive genes in prostate cancer cells, researchers concluded that, "Resveratrol may be a useful chemopreventive/chemotherapeutic agent for prostate cancer." Also, resveratrol reverses increases in PSA in cancer cells. For example, in one study, four days of resveratrol treatment resulted in an **80% reduction** in PSA levels in prostate cancer cells. Resveratrol also modulates growth factors, protects DNA, blocks cancer-causing chemicals and radiation, and fights free radicals and inflammation. The same anticancer gene activated by non-steroidal anti-inflammatory drugs (NSAIDs) demonstrates enhanced expression by resveratrol.

Using a DNA microarray—a scientific research tool that simultaneously examines how particular phytocompounds affect thousands of genes—scientists found that resveratrol exerts a striking effect on cancer-related genes. Among other things, resveratrol activates tumor suppressor genes, other genes that destroy cancer cells, and genes that control the cell cycle—while suppressing genes that allow cancer cells to communicate with one another. This ability to get inside cancer cells and activate or deactivate genes is a powerful weapon against cancer growth—especially since resveratrol exerts its effects without toxicity.

25. BETA-SITOSTEROL

A plant fat and phytosterol known as beta-sito-sterol, used in several European prostate drugs, has been found to block the growth of prostate cancer cells. A study on an androgen-dependent line of prostate cancer cells showed that beta-sitosterol decreased cancer cell growth by **24%** and increased apoptosis **four-fold**. These findings correlated with a **50%** increase in production of ceramide, an important cell membrane component believed to induce apopotosis.

26. GINGER (ZINGIBER OFFICINALE)

A study reported in 2013 demonstrated that ginger phytochemicals work synergistically to inhibit the proliferation of human prostate cancer cells (PC-3 cell line). In past research, ginger showed anti-inflammatory, antioxidant, and antiproliferative activities, suggesting a promising role as a chemopreventive agent. Then, a 2012 study became the first report to clearly demonstrate the anticancer activity of orally taken, whole ginger extract for the therapeutic management of prostate cancer. This breakthrough research found that ginger resulted in growth inhibition, cell-cycle arrest, and induced caspase-dependent intrinsic apoptosis in prostate cancer cells. In vivo studies by this team showed that—without any detectable toxicity—ginger significantly inhibited tumor growth in xenografts of a line of prostate cancer cells (PC3) subcutaneously implanted in nude mice.

Specifically, the scientific team orally fed a solution containing ginger extract to the tumor-implanted mice for eight weeks. Daily measurements of tumor volume were performed. Tumors in control mice that received a placebo solution showed unrestricted growth. But tumors in mice that received the ginger extract solution showed a time-dependent inhibition of growth over the eight-week period. Remarkably, the tumor burden in the ginger group was **reduced** by about **56%** after just eight weeks of feeding. Tumor tissue from ginger extract-treated mice showed a reduced proliferation index and "widespread apoptosis" compared with controls. Ginger treatment was well tolerated, and the test mice maintained normal weight gain and showed no signs of discomfort during the treatment regimen. Most importantly, orally taken ginger extract did not exert any detectable toxicity in normal, rapidly dividing tissues such as the gut and bone marrow.

27. INOSITOL HEXAPHOSPHATE (IP6)

In 2013, scientists designed an IP6 experiment on TRAMP mice, which are genetically modified to develop metastatic prostate cancer. For 24 weeks, mice with prostate cancer were given drinking water that was **0%, 1%, 2%,** or **4%** IP6. The study team periodically conducted magnetic resonance imaging (MRI) tests on each mouse prostate to assess prostate volume and tumor vascularity. The animals that received higher concentrations of IP6 showed a "**profound**" **reduction** in prostate tumor size, due in part to the compound's antiangiogenic effect (the ability of the compound to reduce new blood vessel formation). The researchers discovered a decrease in a glucose transporter protein, known as GLUT-4, in the prostates of IP6-treated mice, and observed that IP6 decreased glucose metabolism and membrane phospholipid synthesis—meaning there was substantial energy deprivation with the tumor itself. This demonstrates "a practical and translational potential of IP6 treatment in suppressing growth and progression of prostate cancer in humans."

28. N-Acetylcysteine (NAC)

NAC inhibited the growth, migration, and invasion of two cell lines (DU145 and PC3 cells). Also, NAC significantly reduced the ability of the prostate cancer cells to attach themselves (to collagen IV-coated surfaces). Inhibition occurred in both cell lines. The team concluded that NAC has high potential to attenuate migration of human prostate cancer cells and to suppress the growth of primary and secondary tumors—and they suggested NAC may represent an affordable and low-toxicity, adjuvant-therapy option for prostate cancer.

J Med Assoc Thai. 2009 Sep;92(9):1171-7.

N-acetylcysteine inhibits proliferation, adhesion, migration and invasion of human bladder cancer cells.

NAC has an anti-metastatic effect on the human bladder cancer cells by inhibiting their growth, adhesion, migration, and invasion properties.

J Med Assoc Thai. 2012 Dec;95 Suppl 12:S56-62.

Antimetastatic potential of N-acetylcysteine on human prostate cancer cells.

NAC could have a high potential in attenuating the migration of the human prostate cancer cells from their primary site and their adhesion and invasion to the remote locations. Hence, NAC might suppress the growth of the primary and the secondary tumors. Our findings suggest that NAC had a high possibility to become an antimetastatic agent for testing in clinical trials. Then, NAC might be used clinically as an optional adjuvant therapeutic drug in addition to the conventional standard treatment of human prostate cancer, obtaining a better outcome with the least toxic and affordable substance

29. BROMELAIN

J Exp Clin Cancer Res. 2014 Nov 12;33:92. doi: 10.1186/s13046-014-0092-7.

Bromelain and N-acetylcysteine inhibit proliferation and survival of gastrointestinal cancer cells in vitro: significance of combination therapy.

We report for the first time to our knowledge the growth-inhibitory and cytotoxic effects of bromelain and N-acetylcysteine, in particular in combination, on a panel of gastrointestinal cancer cell lines with different phenotypes and characteristics. These effects apparently resulted from cell cycle arrest, apoptosis and autophagy. Towards the development of novel strategies for the enhancement of microscopic cytoreduction, our results lay the basis for further evaluation of this formulation in locoregional approaches to peritoneal surface malignancies and carcinomatosis.

Bromelain, an enzyme that can be extracted from pineapple stems, is selectively cytotoxic, and was shown superior to the chemotherapy drug 5-fluorauracil in treating cancer in the animal model

Bromelain is a proteolytic enzyme, which can be helpful in treating cancer because it helps restore balance to your immune system, among other cancer-fighting benefits.

30. QUERCETIN

Lab research has suggested that quercetin inhibits prostate cancer development. Scientists found that quercetin produces a **69% reduction** in the growth of highly aggressive prostate cancer cells, a greater than **50% upregulation** of tumor-suppressor genes, and a **61-100% downregulation** of cancer-promoting oncogenes. A study suggested that quercetin works partially by blocking the androgen receptors used to sustain growth by prostate cancer cells—potentially preventing these cells from forming tumors. Another quercetin anticancer mechanism was revealed in a study on human prostate cancer (PC-3) cells. Quercetin induced the mitochondrial apoptotic signaling pathway and endoplasmic reticulum stress, triggering DNA damage and apoptotic death in these cells. Other research confirmed that quercetin inhibits the migration and invasiveness of prostate cancer cells.

31. REISHI

Constituents called triterpenes in the fungus *Ganoderma lucidum*, better known as reishi mushroom, provide important anti-inflammatory and anti-proliferative effects that play a role in cancer. These mechanisms, combined with the polysaccharides and other components in reishi, can inhibit cancer—including prostate cancer cells. While reishi has been heavily studied for its ability to enhance immunity, some scientists adopted a novel approach to researching potential effects of fungi against prostate cancer. They evaluated the ability of various fungus extracts to act from within the cell to interfere with the androgen receptor and thus, inhibit prostate cancer growth.

These researchers investigated over 200 fungus extracts for their anti-androgenic activity—and of these, *G. lucidum* (reishi) was one of two mushrooms selected for further investigation. This extract also blocked cell proliferation and decreased cancer cell viability. Reishi inhibited androgen-sensitive, human prostate adenocarcinoma cells (LNCaP cells). The published report concluded that, "*G. lucidum* extracts have profound activity against LNCaP cells that merits further investigation as a potential therapeutic agent for the treatment of prostate cancer."

32. 5-Loxin®

Aging humans are at increased risk of health complications and mortality via the upregulation of a proinflammatory enzyme called *5-lipoxygenase*, or *5-LOX*. The 5-LOX enzyme generates a cascade of dangerous inflammatory effects throughout the body—which results in increased vulnerability of the organs to disease and functional deficits, particularly as the aging process progresses. This enzyme stimulates the manufacture of pro-inflammatory molecules called *leukotrienes*, which are linked in abundant research to numerous age-related diseases—including cancer. Compounds in the flowering plant genus *Boswellia*—*beta-boswellic acid*, *keto-beta-boswellic acid*, and *acetyl-keto-beta-boswellic acid (AKBA)*—were shown to induce apoptosis in cancer cells. But a purified extract of *Boswellia* has been specifically shown to selectively inhibit the 5-LOX enzyme.

This purified extract—5-Loxin®—is standardized for AKBA content and protects against inflammatory diseases, including prostate cancer, through several mechanisms. For example, virtually all human cancer cell lines, including prostate cancer cells, induce production of a protein-degrading enzyme called *matrix metalloproteinase (MMP)*, which cancer cells employ to tear apart containment structures within the prostate gland that would normally encase them. This allows the prostate cancer cells to break through healthy prostate tissue and metastasize. However, 5-Loxin® has been shown to prevent expression of MMP—inhibiting the spread of prostate cancer cells.

Prostate cancer cells also use adhesion molecules called *VCAM-1* and *ICAM-1*—which are directly involved in inflammatory processes—to facilitate their spread throughout the body. 5-Loxin® was shown to prevent the up-regulation of these adhesion molecules. Also, the process of angiogenesis that feeds blood to developing cancer tumors is tightly linked to chronic inflammation.

33. GLYCYRRHIZIN

Glycyrrhizin, a triterpene compound isolated from the roots of licorice has been found to exhibit potent *in vitro* cytotoxic activity against both hormone-dependent (LNCaP), and hormone-independent (DU-145), lines of human prostate cancer. In one study, glycyrrhizin inhibited cell proliferation in these cell lines in a time- and dose-dependent manner. The decreased viability was found to be due to apoptosis. Glycyrrhizin also caused DNA damage in these cell lines in a time-dependent manner. This suggests that this licorice compound has therapeutic potential against prostate cancer.

34. MODIFIED CITRUS PECTIN

This modified form has been shown to bind to the important **galectin** molecules on the surface of cells. Scientists believe that this ability of the modified citrus pectin to adhere to molecules—specifically to the **galectin-3 molecule**—is responsible for its demonstrated ability to inhibit cancer cells. This preventive effect was shown in animal research. For example, oral administration of modified citrus pectin inhibited the **spontaneous** extraprostatic **colonization** of injected cells from a prostate cancer cell line and in a dose-dependent fashion.

Cancer cells must communicate with one another to invade, colonize, and proliferate in healthy tissue; but this proprietary citrus pectin appears to disrupt this inter-cellular communication, slowing metastasis. The American Cancer Society suggests that modified citrus pectin may "be useful for preventing or slowing the growth of metastatic tumors in very early stages of development." For instance, **70%** of prostate cancer patients treated orally for 12 months with a modified citrus pectin preparation experienced a slow-down in the rise of **prostate-specific antigen**, or **PSA**, concentrations in the blood—without side effects.

35. APRICOT KERNELS

Amygdalin from apricot kernels induces apoptotic cell death in human DU145 and LNCaP prostate cancer cells. Amygdalin induces apoptotic cell death in human DU145 and LNCaP prostate cancer cells by caspase-3 activation through downregulation of Bcl-2 and upregulation of Bax.

36.   PAU D' ARCO (LA PACHO) TEA

Phosphorylation of p53, induction of Bax and activation of caspases during beta-lapachone-mediated apoptosis in human prostate epithelial cells.

The DNA topoisomerase I inhibitor beta-lapachone, the product of a tree from South America, is known to exhibit various biological properties. The apoptotic effects on human prostate epithelial cells of beta-lapachone were associated with marked induction of p53 phosphorylation and Bax protein without altering the expression of p53 and Bcl-2 protein.

- HepG2 hepatoma cell line through induction of Bax and activation of caspase.

- beta-lapachone induces growth inhibition and apoptosis in bladder cancer cells by modulation of Bcl-2 family and activation of caspases.

37. MELATONIN

Prostate. 2005 Apr 1;63(1):29-43.

Melatonin reduces prostate cancer cell growth leading to neuroendocrine differentiation via a receptor and PKA independent mechanism.

Sainz RM[1], Mayo JC, Tan DX, León J, Manchester L, Reiter RJ.

Abstract

BACKGROUND:

Melatonin, the main secretory product of the pineal gland, inhibits the growth of several types of cancer cells. Melatonin limits human prostate cancer cell growth by a mechanism which involves the regulation of androgen receptor function but it is not clear whether other mechanisms may also be involved.

METHODS:

Time-course and dose-dependent studies were performed using androgen-dependent (LNCaP) and independent (PC3) prostate cancer cells. Cell number, cell viability, and cell cycle progression were studied. Neuroendocrine differentiation of these cells was evaluated by studying morphological and biochemical markers. Finally, molecular mechanisms including the participation of melatonin membrane receptors, intracellular cAMP levels, and the PKA signal transduction pathway were also analyzed.

RESULTS:

Melatonin treatment dramatically reduced the number of prostate cancer cells and stopped cell cycle progression in both LNCaP and PC3 cells. In addition, it induced cellular differentiation as indicated by obvious morphological changes and neuroendocrine biochemical parameters. The role of melatonin in cellular proliferation and differentiation of prostate cancer cells is not mediated by its membrane receptors nor related to PKA activation.

CONCLUSIONS:

The treatment of prostate cancer cells with pharmacological concentrations of melatonin influences not only androgen-sensitive but also androgen-insensitive epithelial prostate cancer cells. Cell differentiation promoted by melatonin is not mediated by PKA activation although it increases, in a transitory manner, intracellular cAMP levels. Melatonin markedly influences the proliferative status of prostate cancer cells. These effects should be evaluated thoroughly since melatonin levels are diminished in aged individuals when prostate cancer typically occurs.

Higher levels of melatonin, a hormone involved in the sleep-wake cycle, may suggest decreased risk for developing advanced prostate cancer, according to results presented at the AACR-Prostate Cancer Foundation Conference on Advances in Prostate Cancer Research, held Jan. 18-21.

Melatonin is a hormone that is produced exclusively at night in the dark and is an important output of the circadian rhythm, or the body's inherent 24-hour clock. Many biological processes are regulated by the circadian rhythm, including the sleep-wake cycle. Melatonin may play a role in regulating a range of other hormones that influence certain cancers, including breast and prostate cancers.

"Sleep loss and other factors can influence the amount of melatonin secretion or block it altogether, and health problems associated with low melatonin, disrupted sleep, and/or disruption of the circadian rhythm are broad, including a potential risk factor for cancer," said Sarah C. Markt, M.P.H., doctoral candidate in the Department of Epidemiology at Harvard School of Public Health in Boston. "We found that men who had higher levels of melatonin had a 75 percent reduced risk for developing advanced prostate cancer compared with men who had lower levels of melatonin.

"Our results require replication, but support the public health implication of the importance of maintaining a stable light-dark and sleep-wake cycle," added Markt. "Because melatonin levels are potentially modifiable, further studies of melatonin and prostate cancer risk and progression are warranted."

To investigate the association between urine levels of the main breakdown product of melatonin, 6-sulfatoxymelatonin, and risk of prostate cancer, Markt and colleagues conducted a case-cohort study of 928 Icelandic men from the AGES-Reykjavik cohort between 2002 and 2009. They collected first morning void urine samples at recruitment, and asked the participants to answer a questionnaire about sleep patterns.

The researchers found that one in seven men reported problems falling asleep, one in five men reported problems staying asleep, and almost one in three reported taking sleeping medications.

The median value of 6-sulfatoxymelatonin in the study participants was 17.14 nanograms per milliliter of urine. Men who reported taking medications for sleep, problems falling asleep, and problems staying asleep had significantly lower 6-sulfatoxymelatonin levels compared with men without sleep problems, according to Markt.

Of the study participants, 111 men were diagnosed with prostate cancer, including 24 with advanced disease. The researchers found that men whose 6-sulfatoxymelatonin levels were higher than the median value had a 75 percent decreased risk for advanced prostate cancer. A 31 percent decreased risk for prostate cancer overall was observed as well, but this finding was not statistically significant.

"Further prospective studies to investigate the interplay between sleep duration, sleep disturbance, and melatonin levels on risk for prostate cancer are needed," said Markt.

From Medscape:

Melatonin and Cancer

Melatonin seems to contribute to cancer prevention and may also be used as additive therapy in cancer.

Melatonin and Protection From Carcinogenesis

Melatonin seems to have an oncostatic action and appears to contribute to anticancer protection [Bukowska, 2011; Hrushesky *et al.* 2009; McCarty, 2012; McCune *et al.* 2011; Mao *et al.* 2010; Mediavilla *et al.* 2010; Ravindra *et al.* 2006; Santoro *et al.* 2012; Schernhammer *et al.* 2011; Vijayalaxmi *et al.* 2002].

Many studies have shown that melatonin inhibits the growth of breast cancer cells, cervical cancer cells and ovarian cancer cells. Melatonin is a new member of a group of regulatory factors controlling cell multiplication and death and is a chronobiotic hormonal regulator of the growth of neoplasmatic cells [Blask *et al.* 2002]. In physiologic concentrations melatonin is cytostatic and inhibits cancer cell multiplication via action in the cell cycle. In pharmacologic concentrations melatonin has a cytotoxic effect on cancer cells. In physiologic and pharmacologic concentrations it acts as a differentiating factor in some cancer cells, reducing their infiltrative and metastatic potential via alteration of binding molecules and conservation of intracellular communication. In other types of cancer cells melatonin either alone or in combination with other factors induces cancer cell apoptosis. Biochemical and molecular mechanisms of the oncostatic action of melatonin include regulation of expression and activation of estrogen receptors *via* calmodulin, modulation of the cytoskeleton architecture and function, and modulation of intracellular oxidative status *via* the cell surface melatonin receptors.

Data show that melatonin inhibits carcinogenesis. Exposure to magnetic fields of 50–60 Hz increases breast cancer risk, possibly via inhibition of melatonin secretion [Liburdy *et al.* 1993]. In rats, having been exposed to the carcinogen 7,12-dimethylbenz[α]anthracene (DMBA), blindness and food restriction prevent the appearance of breast adenocarcinoma, this result being dependent on the presence of the pineal [Bartsch *et al.* 1995]. Food restriction may be related to an increase in melatonin secretion, while blindness leads to the appearance of free rhythms and a strong melatonin signal. This increase seems to be related to an improvement in the natural defense mechanisms of the organism. In rats developing breast cancer after exposure to the carcinogen DMBA, pinealectomy increased the frequency of cancer development while afternoon melatonin administration decreased it.

Indomethacin and melatonin administration inhibits breast cancer development after the administration of DMBA [Mcikova-Kalicka *et al.* 2001]. Melatonin administration in laboratory animals, in which skin carcinogenesis had been induced by benzo-a-pyrene, reduces the number of papillomas in the initiation and progression of carcinogenesis [Kumar and Das, 2000].

Melatonin and Cancer Management

Melatonin may be used as an adjuvant in cancer therapy [Dopfel *et al.* 2007; Han *et al.* 2011; Hansen *et al.* 2012; Jung and Ahmad, 2006; Knower *et al.* 2012; Lissoni *et al.* 1995b, 2001; Lissoni, 2002; Seely *et al.* 2011; Shirazi *et al.* 2007; Srinivasan *et al.* 2011b; Zha *et al.* 2012].

The experimental studies led to clinical studies, in which melatonin was administered along with tamoxifen in women with metastatic breast cancer, which had progressed despite the administration of tamoxifen. It was found that the simultaneous administration of melatonin and tamoxifen may contribute to the objective regression of cancer in women with metastatic breast cancer not responding to tamoxifen alone [Lissoni et al. 1995b].

Studies suggested that the biological response of the host organism to the neoplasm to interleukin 2 may be modulated by the administration of immune-modulating factors, such as melatonin. The parallel administration of melatonin with interleukin 2 in patients with distant metastases in non-small cell lung carcinoma, liver carcinoma, bowel carcinoma, stomach carcinoma, pancreatic carcinoma and breast cancer contributes to cancer regression and disease stabilization [Lissoni et al. 1993].

Melatonin, when used in combination with interleukin 2 in cancer immunotherapy contributes to the prevention of thrombocytopenia, a frequent hematologic complication of interleukin 2 therapy [Lissoni et al. 1995a]. Recent studies have shown that the hemopoietic system is under neuroendocrine control [Lissoni et al. 2001], thrombopoeisis having been shown to be stimulated by melatonin and melatonin shown to be effective in thrombocytopenia therapy.

The number of lymphocytes is one of the most important parameters of the immune system which contribute to the prognosis of patients with progressive cancer. Interleukin 2 and interleukin 12 are the most important cytokines with antineoplastic action in the human organism. The action of these cytokines is modulated by the neuroendocrine system, especially the pineal via the diurnal variation of melatonin secretion [Srinivasan *et al.* 2011b].

The effect of melatonin was investigated in a group of 1440 patients with progressive solid cancer who received supportive therapy with or without melatonin [Lissoni *et al.* 1995b]. The frequency of cachexia, thrombocytopenia and lymphopenia was significantly lower in patients receiving melatonin than in those receiving only supportive therapy. The percentage of patients with disease stabilization and the annual survival were higher in patients receiving melatonin than in those receiving only supportive therapy. The objective response of patients to therapy was significantly greater in patients receiving melatonin and chemotherapy than those receiving only chemotherapy. Melatonin decreased the frequency of cachexia, thrombocytopenia, stomatitis, cardiotoxicity and neurotoxicity due to chemotherapy.

Radiotherapy is a frequent and effective form of cancer therapy. The sensitivity of normal tissues, which are near the neoplasm and are inevitably exposed to radiation, decreases the therapeutic benefit. As ionizing radiation has destructive effects, radiobiologists are interested in the recognition of novel, nontoxic, effective and easy to use methods for the prevention of the damage induced on healthy tissues by radiation. In many studies, melatonin has been proved to decrease the oxidative damage induced by ionizing radiation. Data show that melatonin may be used as a radioprotective agent in patients with cancer either alone for cancer inhibition or in combination with traditional radiotherapy with the aim of a better effectiveness/toxicity ratio [Shirazi *et al.* 2007].

A variety of cytokines and growth factors exert a fine-tuning action in a series of productive and differentiating functions involved in hemopoiesis. Studies have shown that neuroendocrine and neural agents may be involved in the control of hemopoiesis. Melatonin, in particular, may salvage hemopoiesis from the toxic effect of antineoplastic drugs via opioid cytokines of T-helper cells [Maestroni, 1999a].

These studies show that melatonin may be used successfully in clinical oncology as supportive therapy in patients with progressive cancer and for the prevention of toxicity induced by chemotherapy and radiotherapy [Jung and Ahmad, 2006; Dopfel *et al.* 2007]. In conclusion, melatonin may contribute to the protection of organisms from carcinogenesis, being involved in cancer prevention, and may be used as an adjuvant in cancer therapy.

38. SPICES VS. CANCER

Turmeric/Curcumin: Turmeric contains the powerful polyphenol Curcumin that has been clinically proven to retard the growth of cancer cells causing prostate cancer, melanoma, breast cancer, brain tumor, pancreatic cancer and leukemia amongst a host of others. Curcumin promotes 'Apoptosis'- (programmed cell death/cell suicide) that safely eliminates cancer breeding cells without posing a threat to the development of other healthy cells. In cases of conventional radiotherapy and chemotherapy, the surrounding cells too become a target in addition to the cancer cells. Therefore, the side-effects are imminent.

Fennel: Packed with phytonutrients and antioxidants, 'Anethole', a major constituent of fennel resists and restricts the adhesive and invasive activities of cancer cells. It suppresses the enzymatic regulated activities behind cancer cell multiplication.

Saffron: A natural carotenoid dicarboxylic acid called 'Crocetin' is the primary cancer-fighting element that saffron contains. It not only inhibits the progression of the disease but also decreases the size of the tumor by half. Crocetin affects the growth of cancer cells by inhibiting nucleic acid synthesis, enhancing anti-oxidative system, inducing apoptosis and hindering growth factor signaling pathways.

Cumin: A portent herb with anti-oxidant characteristics, cumin seeds contain a compound called 'Thymoquinone' that checks proliferation of cells responsible for prostate cancer.

Cinnamon: It takes no more than a half teaspoon of cinnamon powder every day to keep cancer risk away. A natural food preservative, cinnamon is a source of iron and calcium. Useful in reducing tumor growth, it blocks the formation of new vessels in the human body.

Oregano: More than a pizza or pasta topping, oregano confirms its worth as a potential agent against prostate cancer. Consisting of anti-microbial compounds, just one teaspoon of oregano has the power of two cups of red grapes! Phytochemical 'Quercetin' present in oregano restricts growth of malignant cells in the body and acts like a drug against cancer-centric diseases.

Cayenne Pepper/Capsaicin (Chili peppers): A promising spice with anti-cancer properties. Capsaicin induces the process of apoptosis that destroys potential cancer cells and reduces the size of leukemia tumor cells considerably.

Ginger: This humble spice boasts of medicinal qualities that help lowering cholesterol, boost metabolism and kill cancer cells. Details above.

Others: Cloves, anise, basil, garlic, caraway, fenugreek, mustard, mint leaves, rosemary, Limonin (fresh lemon), virgin olive, vinegar and avocado are other cancer-fighting diet components.

39. URSOLIC ACID

Ursolic acid, a naturally occurring triterpenoid, demonstrates anticancer activity on human prostate cancer cells

Results

Ursolic acid inhibited significantly the cell viability and induced apoptosis in PC-3 cells at 55 µM and in LNCaP cells at 45 µM associated with a down regulation of bcl-2 protein.

Conclusions

The antiproliferative and apoptotic effects of ursolic acid in PC-3 and LNCaP cells implicate its potential therapeutic use for the treatment of hormone refractory and androgen-sensitive prostate cancer. The down regulation of bcl-2 may be one of the molecular mechanisms via which it induces apoptosis in PC-3 and LNCaP cells.

Animal studies have found benefits with ursolic acid in the diet at 0.05-0.2% of the diet, which is around 10-40mg/kg (based on their weight and food intake) and the estimated human dose equivalent to this is 1.6-6.4mg/kg bodyweight; for a 150lb adult it would be the range of 110-440mg.

Apoptotic action of ursolic acid isolated from Corni fructus in RC-58T/h/SA#4 primary human prostate cancer cells

Abstract

Ursolic acid (3β-hydroxy-urs-12-en-28-oic acid) is a major biological active component of Corni fructus that is known to induce apoptosis. However, the apoptotic mechanism of ursolic acid using primary malignant tumor (RC-58T/h/SA#4)-derived human prostate cells is not known. In the present study, ursolic acid significantly inhibited the growth of RC-58T/h/SA#4 cells in dose- and time-dependent manners. Ursolic acid induced cell death as evidenced by an increased proportion of cells in sub-G1 phase, the formation of apoptotic bodies, nuclear condensation, and DNA fragmentation. After ursolic acid treatment at concentrations above 40 µM, the activities of caspase-3, -8, and -9 were significantly increased compared that of control. Ursolic acid modulated the upregulation of Bax (pro-apoptotic) as well as the down regulation of Bcl-2 (anti-apoptotic). Ursolic acid also stimulated Bid cleavage, which indicates that the apoptotic action of caspase-8-mediated Bid cleavage leads to the activation of caspase-9. Thus, the apoptotic effect of ursolic acid was involved in extrinsic and intrinsic signaling pathways. In addition, ursolic acid increased the expression of the caspase-independent mitochondrial apoptosis factor (AIF) in RC-58T/h/SA#4 cells. The present results suggest that ursolic acid from Corni fructus activated apoptosis in RC-58T/h/SA#4 cells via both caspase-dependent and -independent pathways.

40. TRT, ESTROGEN/PROGESTERONE

From: http://elitemensguide.com/testosterone-levels-by-age/

Testosterone Levels by Age: The BAD News

As You Age:

Total
Testosterone
Levels

Free
Testosterone
Levels

As men age, total testosterone levels decline. Even worse, free testosterone (testosterone not bound in the blood to sex hormone-binding globulin (SHBG)) levels decline more rapidly than total testosterone. Studies have shown that total testosterone decreases by approximately 30% in healthy men between the ages of 25 and 75. Free testosterone levels decline even more significantly with decreases of approximately 50%.

The official term for this decline is Late Onset Hypogonadism (LOH) also known as andropause, but it's more commonly referred to as low testosterone or, simply, "Low T". The following table by A. Vermeleun (1996) shows total testosterone levels by age as well as

Age	Total Testosterone (ng/dl)	Free Testosterone (ng/dl)	SHBG (nmol/L)
25-34	617	12.3	35.5
35-44	668	10.3	40.1
45-54	606	9.1	44.6
55-64	562	8.3	45.5
65-74	524	6.9	48.7
75-84	471	6.0	51
85-100	376	5.4	65.9

free testosterone levels and SHBG levels. As you can see, total testosterone declines with aging. Also, the amount of SHBG increases with aging causing the much more dramatic drop in free testosterone.

What Problems Result From Low Testosterone?

Low testosterone has been correlated with unwanted changes in body composition such as increased abdominal fat and decreased muscle mass. Unfortunately, abdominal fat affects organs like the heart, liver and kidneys more adversely than fat anywhere else, in terms of cardiovascular risk. Unsurprisingly, low testosterone levels by age are associated with an increased risk of cardiovascular disease and metabolic problems, such as diabetes. Low testosterone can also cause erectile dysfunction, depression, mood changes, and low bone density.

Testosterone Levels by Age: The GOOD News

Fortunately, certain healthy lifestyle choices, such as exercise and proper diet, may actually increase testosterone production naturally. Additionally, the simple hormone treatment of testosterone, known as **Testosterone Replacement Therapy (TRT),** for men with low testosterone can improve many symptoms associated with low T including sexual function, muscle mass and strength, body composition, and bone density, and may also benefit other critical functions including metabolic, cardiovascular, and cognitive function.

Unfortunately, most primary care physicians and some endocrinologists don't know how to recognize or treat hypogonadism. The right blood tests are essential starting with total and free testosterone. I have tested many men to find normal total testosterone and very low free testosterone. Free testosterone is the component that has all the health benefits. Fenugreek can raise free testosterone. After one month of Testosterone Replacement Therapy estradiol, progesterone, PSA, free and total testosterone should be checked.

Conversion factor: 1 ng/ml = 3.18 nmol/l

Normal male progesterone level should be above 0.1 and closer to 1.0 ng/ml

Symptoms of low progesterone in men include:

- Bone loss
- Depression
- Erectile dysfunction
- Fatigue
- Gynecomastia ("man-boobs")
- Hair loss
- Impotence·
- Low libido
- Muscle loss
- Weight gain

Known Problems with Estrogen Dominance:

- Cellular changes leading to cancer, including breast cancer in men
- Depression and fatigue
- Enlargement of the prostate
- Erectile dysfunction
- Excess, stubborn and hard to lose body fat, especially abdominal and chest fat
- Gynecomastia (man boobs)
- Hair loss
- Heart disease (makes you more prone to chest pains and heart attacks)
- Increased frequency of urination (waking up multiple times at night to go for a pee)
- Inflammation of the prostate
- Male breast tenderness
- Reduced sex-drive

Known Benefits of Natural Progesterone Therapy:

- Corrects erectile dysfunction in much the way Viagra does, by increasing production of nitric oxide
- Diminishes muscular aches and pains, has anti-inflammatory properties
- Helps normalize blood sugar levels
- Helps use fat for energy, making it easier to lose weight
- Improves brain function, has antidepressant properties
- Improves skin problems including acne, seborrhea, rosacea, psoriasis
- Improves sleep pattern
- Increases muscle mass
- Increases sexual drive
- Normalizes thyroid hormone function
- Protects against prostate and breast cancer (both are increasing in men)
- Stimulates new bone formation

41. MY PERSONAL JOURNEY

My PSA went from a consistent (4.5 + or - 0.2) to 7.47 in 17 mos. I was treated with several antibiotics thinking it was prostatitis then it went to 9.89 in two mos. I postponed my next urologic appointment because I was scared it is probably prostate cancer. That is when I began my research. I was already eating healthful (I thought) and taking many vitamins and supplements. My urologist scheduled me for a prostate biopsy. I began adding nutrients to my program and continued to discover more to add. My PSA dropped to 6.3 in two mos. and to 4.2 in another mo. 3.64 in two more months. This was lower than it was six years ago. I cancelled my biopsy. Here is my program:

42. NATURAL CHEMOTHERAPY FOR PROSTATE CANCER

Discuss this program with your doctor who understands natural treatment and possible interactions with medications. Consultations in person, phone, text or email with me can be scheduled at (606) 324-3668 must be prepaid.

1. Super MiraForte with Standardized Lignans and ProstaPollen™ from LEF.org

2. Beet root powder start with one tablespoon then double in two weeks.

3. 5-Loxin® is 50-100 milligrams daily with or without food. Individuals with prostate cancer may consider dosages of 150 to 250 milligrams a day of 5-Loxin®.

4. Grape seed extract 300 milligrams daily.

5. Glycyrrhizin.

6. Modified Citrus Pectin 15 grams between meals.

7. Boron is 1-8 milligrams daily.

8. Daily suggested dosages are 14 milligrams for DIM, and 80-160 milligrams for I3C. An I3C dosage of 200-600 milligrams daily is suggested as an adjuvant for prostate cancer therapy. Watercress extract is 50-100 milligrams daily, taken with or without food. Dosages for PEITC are not well-

established. I take Triple Action Cruciferous Vegetable Extract 3 times a day.

9. Apigenin 100 mg daily

10. Soy isoflavones is 135-270 milligrams daily with food or eat edamame two servings daily.

11. Vit D 10,000 daily.

12. EGCG 3,000 milligrams.

13. Omega-3 Fatty Acids 8 grams daily.

14. Curcumin. 800-1,200 milligrams daily with food.

15. Co-Q 10 500 milligrams daily, both taken after a meal.

16. Gamma-Tocopherol Vitamin E 1000 iu daily. I take Gamma E Tocopherol with Sesame Lignans from LEF.org

17. Lycopene 45 milligrams daily with food.

18. Selenium 200 micrograms daily.

19. Standardized milk thistle extract is 750 milligrams daily , taken with or without food.

20. Zinc 50mg not sulfate.

21. GLA dosage 700-900 milligrams daily, with meals.

22. Zeaxanthin 3.75 milligrams daily.

23. Pomegranate 280-375 milligrams daily (of punicalagins), with or without food. I take Endothelial Defense™ with Full-Spectrum Pomegranate™ from LEF.org and pomegranate powder and juice.

24. Saw palmetto is 320 milligrams daily.

25. Resveratrol, the suggested dosage is 20-250 milligrams a day, taken with or without food. I take Optimized Resveratrol with NAD+ Cell Regenerator™ from LEF.org

26. Lignands 75-125 milligrams daily 4 to 6 tablespoons of ground organic flax seed daily.

27. Vitamin K2 1,000 micrograms for the menaquinone-4 form of K2 (MK-4) and 200 micrograms for the menaquinone-7 (MK-7) form.

28. Beta-sitosterol 169 mg twice daily.

29. Ginger extract was found to be approximately 567 milligrams daily for a 154-pound (70 kilogram) human adult.

30. Inositol Hexaphosphate (IP6) 10 grams.

31. N-Acetylcysteine (NAC) 1,200 daily.

32. Quercetin 1,000 to 3,000 mg daily.

33. Reishi extract is 3000 milligrams daily I take Immune Senescence Protection Formula™ from LEF.org

34. Bromelain up to 2000 milligrams daily in divided doses.

35. Black cumin seed oil. 1 tsp once or twice daily.

36. NK cell activator. Proprietary Enzymatically Modified Rice Bran 500.

43. DIETARY INTERVENTION TO ENHANCE IMMUNITY

Because more than half of your immune system is in your gut diet and bacterial flora are extremely important. The average human has 6 pounds of bacteria in their bowels. More bacterial cells than human cells in the whole body.

The best diet, is whole food vegan or at least minimize the animal products.

Prebiotics. These promote healthy flora. As you will note, the best options are raw foods.

1. Raw asparagus
2. Raw chicory root
3. Raw dandelion greens
4. Raw garlic
5. Raw Jerusalem artichoke
6. Raw leeks
7. Raw onion

Probiotic Foods. These have healthful bacteria.

1. Cheeses (organic from grass fed cows)
2. Kefir

3. Kimchi
4. Sauerkraut
5. Tempeh
6. Tofu

A Healthy Approach to "Detox"

1. Eliminate processed food
2. Choose purified alkalinized water
3. Increase your water consumption
4. Carefully choose your supplements, choose those based on real, whole foods
5. Select organic foods

Key Ways to Boost and Rebuild Your Immune System

1. Eliminate processed food
2. Eliminate junk food, including diet and regular soft drinks and soda
3. Dramatically reduce or eliminate sugar
4. Eliminate all artificial sweeteners except stevia in moderation
5. Eliminate trans fats (except conjugated linoleic acid, CLA)
6. Eliminate polyunsaturated fat (these turn into trans fats with cooking and exposure to oxygen..
7. Consume healthy fats like extra virgin olive oil, organic coconut oil, avocado oil, macadamia oil
8. Eat raw foods, such as fruits, vegetables and raw nuts

9. Opt for organic food options when available
10. Consider adopting a gluten free diet
11. Consider grain alternatives such as listed below
12. Don't assume that everything labeled "organic" or "gluten-free" is healthful
13. Eat omega-3 rich foods
14. When possible take supplements that are based on whole foods
15. Pay special attention to the quality of your protein choices
16. Eat foods that fight inflammation, such as turmeric and ginger
17. Eat raw foods more difficult to digest cooked foods especially animal foods
18. Get enough sleep 7 to 9 hours
19. Meditate and stay in touch with yourself through journaling
20. Exercise 25 mins 6 days a week
21. Maintain your waist circumference at the belly button to less than 1/2 your height in inches.
22. Stop smoking
23. Moderate alcohol consumption best are red wine and dark beers.
24. Consume foods rich in prebiotics and probiotics
25. Drink purified water alkalinized.
26. Take steps to purify your air and water
27. Discover your food sensitivities
28. Listen to your body and respond accordingly
29. Read my book **Secrets to Happiness, Inner Peace and Health** to learn more about emotional and spiritual health

44. Top 100 Healthiest Foods

as found on: http://www.whfoods.com/foodstoc.php

Vegetables

Asparagus	Green beans
Avocados	Green peas
Beet greens	Kale
Beets	Leeks
Bell peppers	Mushrooms, crimini
Bok choy	Mushrooms, shiitake
Broccoli	Mustard greens
Brussels sprouts	Olive oil, extra virgin
Cabbage	Olives
Carrots	Onions
Cauliflower	Potatoes
Celery	Romaine lettuce
Collard greens	Sea vegetables
Corn	Spinach
Cucumbers	Squash, summer
Eggplant	Squash, winter
Fennel	Sweet potatoes
Garlic	Swiss chard

Tomatoes	Turnip	greens

Fruits

Apples	Lemon/Limes
Apricots	Oranges
Bananas	Papaya
Blueberries	Pears
Cantaloupe	Pineapple
Cranberries	Plums & Prunes
Figs	Raspberries
Grapefruit	Strawberries
Grapes	Watermelon
Kiwifruit	

Seafood

Cod

Salmon (wild caught not farm raised)

Sardines (low sodium in extra virgin olive oil)

Scallops

Shrimp

Tuna (light not white)

Nuts & Seeds (raw not roasted or salted are preferred)

Almonds

Cashews

Flaxseeds (grind your own)

Peanuts

Pumpkin seeds

Sesame seeds

Sunflower seeds

Walnuts

Beans & Legumes

Black beans

Dried peas

Garbanzo beans (chickpeas)

Kidney beans

Lentils

Lima beans

Miso

Navy beans

Pinto beans

Soy sauce

Soybeans

Tempeh

Tofu

Poultry & Meats

Beef, grass-fed

Chicken, pasture-raised

Lamb, grass-fed

Turkey, pasture-raised

Eggs & Dairy

Cheese, grass-fed

Cow's milk, grass-fed

Eggs, pasture-raised

Yogurt, grass-fed

Grains

Barley

Brown rice

Buckwheat

Millet

Oats

Quinoa

Rye

Whole wheat (not if you are overweight or have waist circumference greater than ½ your height all in inches))

World's Healthiest Herbs & Spices

Basil

Black pepper

Chili pepper, dried

Cilantro & Coriander seeds

Cinnamon, ground

Cloves

Cumin seeds

Dill

Ginger

Mustard seeds

Oregano

Parsley

Peppermint

Rosemary

Sage

Thyme

Turmeric

45

CHARACTERISTICS OF HUMAN PROSTATE CANCER AND IMMORTALIZED CELL LINES

Cell line	Androgen receptor	Androgen sensitivity	5α-Reductase
PC-93	?	AI	–
PC-3	–	AI	–
DU-145	–	AI	–
TSU-Pr1	–	AI	NR
LNCaP	+	AS	–
	Mutated		
Sublines:			
C4	AI	++	
C4-2	AI + mets	+++	+
C4-2B	AI + mets	+++	+
P104-R2 Stimulated			
by finasteride			
LN3		Less sensitive	+++
		than LNCaP	
MDA Prostate cancer 2a	+	AS	
MDA Prostate cancer 2b	+	AS	
ALVA101	+	AS	+
22Rv1	Grown from an	AS	NR
	AI xenograft		
ARCaP	+	Androgen repressed	NR
LACP-4	+	AS	NR
P69SV40T	NR	NR	NR
RWPE-2	+ +	NR	
CA-HPV-10	NR	NR	NR

aNR, not reported.

118

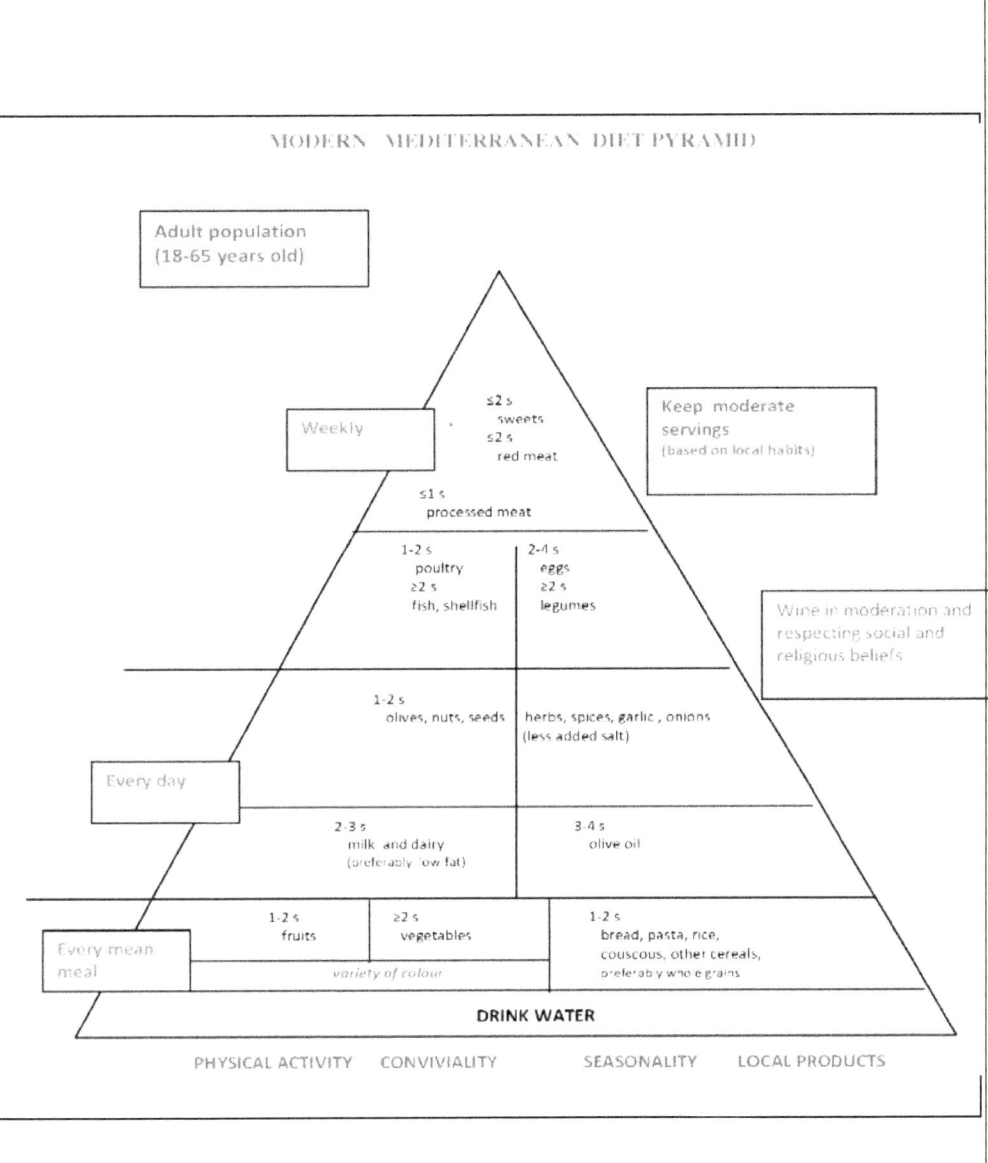

MODERN MEDITERRANEAN DIET PYRAMID

Adult population
(18-65 years old)

Weekly

≤2 s
sweets
≤2 s
red meat

Keep moderate
servings
(based on local habits)

≤1 s
processed meat

1-2 s
poultry
≥2 s
fish, shellfish

2-4 s
eggs
≥2 s
legumes

Wine in moderation and
respecting social and
religious beliefs

1-2 s
olives, nuts, seeds

herbs, spices, garlic , onions
(less added salt)

Every day

2-3 s
milk and dairy
(preferably low fat)

3-4 s
olive oil

Every meal meal

1-2 s
fruits

≥2 s
vegetables

1-2 s
bread, pasta, rice,
couscous, other cereals,
preferably whole grains

variety of colour

DRINK WATER

PHYSICAL ACTIVITY   CONVIVIALITY   SEASONALITY   LOCAL PRODUCTS

ABOUT THE AUTHOR

Dr. Brian K. Bailey is a Podiatric Physician & Surgeon a foot specialist. **Body-Mind-Spirit Podiatric Center** is located in downtown Ashland, KY at the corner of 14th Street and Central Avenue.

Dr. Bailey is a graduate of the University of California at Davis, graduating with a Bachelor of Science in Physiology in 1982 afterwards completing a year of graduate work in education. Continuing his education, he graduated from California College of Podiatric Medicine where he received a Bachelor of Science in Basic Medical Science in 1985 and Doctor of Podiatric Medicine in 1987.

Dr. Bailey has been an Adjunct Professor employed with Ashland Community College teaching anatomy & physiology. Dr. Bailey is also Clinical Professor of Podiatric Medicine and Surgery at Pikeville College, School of Osteopathic Medicine. He has students and residents rotating through his office. After the publication of his book in 1997, "**Secrets to Happiness, Inner Peace and Health**," he continues to give health consults on diet, fitness, and supplements for natural healing, weight loss and rejuvenation. His last book is BREAST CANCER PREVENTION AND WHOLISTIC TREATMENT: NATURAL NON-TOXIC CHEMOTHERAPY FOR BREAST CANCER

Before that "**Metabolic Syndrome 2011**".

References:

1. Aggarwal BB, Bhardwaj A, Aggarwal RS, Seeram NP, Shishodia S, Takada Y. Role of resveratrol in prevention and therapy of cancer: preclinical and clinical studies. *Anticancer Res.* 2004 Sep-Oct;24(5A):2783-840.

2. Aggarwal BB, Sundaram C, Malani N, Ichikawa H. Curcumin: the Indian solid gold. *Adv Exp Med Biol.* 2007;595:1-75.

3. Albertsen K, Gronbaek M. Does amount or type of alcohol influence the risk of prostate cancer? *Prostate.* 2002;52:297-304.

4. Angelucci A, Garofalo S, Speca S, et al. Arachidonic acid modulates the crosstalk between prostate carcinoma and bone stromal cells. *Endocr Relat Cancer.* 2008 Mar;15(1):91-100.

5. Antony B, Merina B, Iyer VS, Judy N, Lennertz K, Joyal S. A pilot cross-over study to evaluate human oral bioavailability of BCM-95CG (Biocurcumax); A novel bioenhanced preparation of curcumin. *Indian J Pharm Sci.* 2008 Jul-Aug;70(4):445-9.

6. Awad AB, Burr AT, Fink CS. Effect of resveratrol and beta-sitosterol in combination on reactive oxygen species and prostaglandin release by PC-3 cells. *Prostaglandins Leukot Essent Fatty Acids.* 2005 Mar;72(3):219-26.

7. Awad AB, Fink CS, Williams H, Kim U. In vitro and in vivo (SCID mice) effects of phytosterols on the growth and dissemination of human prostate cancer PC-3 cells. *Eur J Cancer Prev.* 2001 Dec;10(6):507-13.

8. Baek SJ, Wilson LC, Eling TE. Resveratrol enhances the expression of nonsteroidal anti-inflammatory drug-activated gene (NAG-1) by increasing the expression of p53. *Carcinogenesis.* 2002 Mar;23(3):425-34.

9. Barranco WT, Eckhert CD. Boric acid inhibits human prostate cancer cell proliferation. *Cancer Lett.* 2004 Dec 8;216(1):21-9.

10. Bataineh ZM, Hani IH Bani, Al-Alami JR. Zinc in normal and pathological human prostate gland. *Saudi Med Jour.* 2002;23(2):218-20.

11. Beaver LM, Yu TW, Sokolowski EI, Williams DE, Dashwood RH, Ho E. 3,3'-Diindolylmethane, but not indole-3-carbinol, inhibits histone deacetylase activity in prostate cancer cells. *Toxicol Appl Pharmacol.* 2012 Sep 15;263(3):345-51.

12. Bergman JM, Thompson LU, Dabrosin C. Flaxseed and its lignans inhibit estradiol-induced growth, angiogenesis, and secretion of vascular endothelial growth factor in human breast cancer xenografts in vivo. *Clin Cancer Res.* 2007 Feb 1;13(3):1061-7.

13. Bergman Jungeström M, Thompson LU, Dabrosin C. Flaxseed and its lignans inhibit estradiol-induced growth, angiogenesis, and secretion of vascular endothelial growth factor in human breast cancer xenografts in vivo. *Clin Cancer Res.* 2007 Feb 1;13(3):1061-7.

14. Bettuzzi S, Brausi M, Rizzi F, Castagnetti G, Peracchia G, Corti A. Chemoprevention of human prostate cancer by oral administration of green tea catechins in volunteers with high-grade prostate intraepithelial neoplasia: a preliminary report from a one-year proof-of-principle study. *Cancer Res.* 2006 Jan 15;66(2):1234-40.

15. Billis A. Latent carcinoma and atypical lesions of prostate. An autopsy study. *Urology.* 1986 Oct;28(4):324-9.

16. Bonkhoff H, Fixemer T. Implications of estrogens and their receptors for the development and progression of prostate cancer. *Pathologe.* 2005 Nov;26(6):461-8.

17. Brahmbhatt M, Gundala SR, Asif G, Shamsi SA, Aneja R. Ginger phytochemicals exhibit synergy to inhibit prostate cancer cell proliferation. *Nutr Cancer.* 2013 Feb;65(2):263-72.

18. Brasky TM, Kristal AR, Navarro SL, et al. Specialty supplements and prostate cancer risk in the VITamins and Lifestyle (VITAL) cohort. *Nutr Cancer .* 2011;63(4):573-82.

19. Brooks JD, Metter EJ, Chan DW, et al. Plasma selenium level before diagnosis and the risk of prostate cancer development. *J Urol.* 2001 Dec;166(6):2034-8.

20. Chao C, Haque R, Van Den Eeden SK, Caan BJ, Poon KY, et al. Red wine consumption and risk of prostate cancer: the California men's health study. *Int J Cancer.* 2010;126:171-9.

21. Chaudhary LR, Hruska KA. Inhibition of cell survival signal protein kinase B/Akt by curcumin in human prostate cancer cells. *J Cell Biochem.* 2003;89(1):1-5.

22. Chen LH, Fang J, Li H, Demark-Wahnefried W, Lin X. Enterolactone induces apoptosis in human prostate carcinoma LNCaP cells via a mitochondrial-mediated, caspase-dependent pathway. *Mol Cancer Ther.* 2007 Sep;6(9):2581-90.

23. Chen LH, Fang J, Sun Z, Li H, Wu Y, Demark-Wahnefried W, Lin X. Enterolactone inhibits insulin-like growth factor-1 receptor signaling in human prostatic carcinoma PC-3 cells. *J Nutr.* 2009 Apr;139(4):653-9.

24. Chiao JW, Wu H, Ramaswamy G, et al. Ingestion of an isothiocyanate metabolite from cruciferous vegetables inhibits growth of human prostate cancer cell xenografts by apoptosis and cell cycle arrest. *Carcinogenesis.* 2004 Aug;25(8):1403-8.

25. Chinni SR, Li Y, Upadhyay S, Koppolu PK, Sarkar FH. Indole-3-carbinol (I3C) induced cell growth inhibition, G1 cell cycle arrest and apoptosis in prostate cancer cells. *Oncogene.* 2001 May 24;20(23):2927-36.

26. Chinnici CM, Yao Y, Pratico D. The 5-lipoxygenase enzymatic pathway in the mouse brain: young versus old. *Neurobiol Aging.* 2007 Sep;28(9):1457-62.

27. Choi HY, Lim JE, Hong JH. Curcumin interrupts the interaction between the androgen receptor and Wnt/beta-catenin signaling pathway

in LNCaP prostate cancer cells. *Prostate Cancer Prostatic Dis.* 2010 Dec;13(4):343-9.

28. Christen S, Woodall AA, Shigenaga MK, Southwell-Keely PT, Duncan MW, Ames BN. Gamma-tocopherol traps mutagenic electrophiles such as NO(X) and complements alpha-tocopherol: physiological implications. *Proc Natl Acad Sci U S A.* 1997 Apr 1;94(7):3217-22.

29. Chu J, Pratico D. The 5-lipoxygenase as a common pathway for pathological brain and vascular aging. *Cardiovasc Psychiatry Neurol.* 2009;2009:174657.

30. Clark LC, Combs GF, Jr., Turnbull BW. et al. Effects of selenium supplementation for cancer prevention in patients with carcinoma of the skin. A randomized controlled trial. Nutritional Prevention of Cancer Study Group. *JAMA.* 1996;276:1957-63.

31. Clark LC, Dalkin B, Krongrad A, et al. Decreased incidence of prostate cancer with selenium supplementation: results of a double-blind cancer prevention trial. *Br J Urol.* 1998 May;81(5):730-4.

32. Cooney RV, Franke AA, Harwood PJ, Hatch-Pigott V, Custer LJ, Mordan LJ. a-Tocopherol detoxification of nitrogen dioxide: Superiority to a-tocopherol. *Proc Natl Acad Sci USA.* 1993;90(5):1771–1775.

33. Cui Y, Winton MI, Zhang ZF, et al. Dietary boron intake and prostate cancer risk. *Oncol Rep.* 2004 Apr;11(4):887-92.

34. Cytotoxic effect of the red beetroot (Beta vulgaris L.) extract compared to doxorubicin (Adriamycin) in the human prostate (PC-3) and breast (MCF-7) cancer cell lines. Anticancer Agents Med Chem. 2011 Mar;11(3):280-4.Kapadia GJ[1], Azuine MA, Rao GS, Arai T, Iida A, Tokuda H.

35. Davis-Searles PR, Nakanishi Y, Kim NC, et al. Milk thistle and prostate cancer: differential effects of pure flavonolignans from Silybum marianum on antiproliferative end points in human prostate carcinoma cells. *Cancer Res.* 2005 May 15;65(10):4448-57.

36. Demark-Wahnefried W, Polascik TJ, et al. Flaxseed supplementation (not dietary fat restriction) reduces prostate cancer proliferation rates in men presurgery. *Cancer Epidemiol Biomarkers Prev.* 2008 Dec;17(12):3577-87.

37. Demark-Wahnefried W, Robertson CN, Walther PJ, Polascik TJ, Paulson DF, Vollmer RT. Pilot study to explore effects of low-fat, flaxseed-supplemented diet on proliferation of benign prostatic epithelium and prostate-specific antigen. *Urology.* 2004 May;63(5):900-4.

38. Dias VC, Parsons HG. Modulation in delta 9, delta 6, and delta 5 fatty acid desaturase activity in the human intestinal CaCo-2 cell line. *J Lipid Res.* 1995 Mar;36(3):552-63.

39. Donaldson MS. Nutrition and cancer: a review of the evidence for an anti-cancer diet. *Nutr J.* 2004 Oct 20;3:19.

40. Dorai T, Cao YC, Dorai B, Buttyan R, Katz AE. Therapeutic potential of curcumin in human prostate cancer. III. Curcumin inhibits proliferation, induces apoptosis, and inhibits angiogenesis of LNCaP prostate cancer cells in vivo. *Prostate*. 2001;47(4):293-303.

41. du Toit PJ, van Aswegen CH, du Plessis DJ. The effect of essential fatty acids on growth and urokinase-type plasminogen activator production in human prostate DU-145 cells. *Prostaglandins Leukot Essent Fatty Acids*. 1996;55:173-7.

42. Duan RD. Anticancer compounds and sphingolipid metabolism in the colon. *In Vivo*. 2005 Jan-Feb;19(1):293-300.

43. Dubuisson JG, Dyess DL, Gaubatz JW. Resveratrol modulates human mammary epithelial cell O-acetyltransferase, sulfo transferase, and kinase activation of the het- erocyclic amine carcinogen N-hydroxy-PhIP. *Cancer Lett*. 2002 Aug 8;182(1):27-32.

44. Dudhgaonkar S, Thyagarajan A, Sliva D. Suppression of the inflammatory response by triterpenes isolated from the mushroom Ganoderma lucidum. *Int Immunopharmacol*. 2009 Oct;9(11):1272-80.

45. Duffield-Lillico, AJ, Reid, ME, Turnbull, BW, et al. Baseline characteristics and the effect of selenium supplementation on cancer incidence in a randomized clinical trial: a summary report of the Nutritional Prevention of Cancer Trial. *Cancer Epidemiol. Biomarkers Prev*. 2002;11:630-9.

46. Eichholzer M, Steinbrecher A, Kaaks R, et al. Effects of selenium status, dietary glucosinolate intake and serum glutathione s-transferase a activity on the risk of benign prostatic hyperplasia. *BJU Int*. 2012 Dec;110(11 Pt C):E879-85.

47. El-Bayoumy K. The negative results of the SELECT study do not necessarily discredit the selenium-cancer prevention hypothesis. *Nutr Cancer*. 2009;61(3):285-6.

48. El-Sayed WM, Aboul-Fadl T, Lamb JG, Roberts JC, Franklin MR. Effect of selenium-containing compounds on hepatic chemoprotective enzymes in mice. *Toxicology*. 2006 Mar 15;220(2-3):179-88.

49. Evans BA, Griffiths K, Morton MS. Inhibition of 5 alpha-reductase in genital skin fibroblasts and prostate tissue by dietary lignans and isoflavonoids. *J Endocrinol*. 1995 Nov;147(2):295-302.

50. Fang J, Xia C, Cao Z, Zheng JZ, Reed E, Jiang BH. Apigenin inhibits VEGF and HIF-1 expression via PI3K/AKT/p70S6K1 and HDM2/p53 pathways. *FASEB J*. 2005 Mar;19(3):342-53.

51. Fang J, Zhou Q, Liu LZ, et al. Apigenin inhibits tumor angiogenesis through decreasing HIF-1alpha and VEGF expression. *Carcinogenesis*. 2007 Apr;28(4):858-64.

52. Farhan H, Wahala K, Adlercreutz H, et al. Isoflavonoids inhibit catabolism of vitamin D in prostate cancer cells. *J Chromatogr B Analyt Technol Biomed Life Sci*. 2002 Sep 25;777(1-2):261-8.

53. Faronato M, Muzzonigro G, Milanese G, et al. Increased expression of 5-lipoxygenase is common in clear cell renal cell carcinoma. *Histol Histopathol.* 2007 Oct;22(10):1109-18.
54. Fleshner N, Fair WR, Huryk R. et al. Vitamin E inhibits the high-fat diet promoted growth of established human prostate LNCaP tumors in nude mice. *J Urol.* 1999;161:1651-4.
55. Folkers K, Brown R, Judy WV, Morita M. Survival of cancer patients on therapy with coenzyme Q10. *Biochem Biophys Res Commun.* 1993 Apr 15;192(1):241-5.
56. Folkers K, Osterborg A, Nylander M, Morita M, Mellstedt H. Activities of vitamin Q10 in animal models and a serious deficiency in patients with cancer. *Biochem Biophys Res Commun.* 1997 May 19;234(2):296-9.
57. Folkers K. Relevance of the biosynthesis of coenzyme Q10 and of the four bases of DNA as a rationale for the molecular causes of cancer and a therapy. *Biochem Biophys Res Commun.* 1996 Jul 16;224(2):358-61.
58. Fong AT, Swanson HI, Dashwood RH, Williams DE, Hendricks JD, Bailey GS. Mechanisms of anti-carcinogenesis by indole-3-carbinol. Studies of enzyme induction, eletrophile-scavenging, and inhibition of aflatoxin B1 activation. *Biochem Pharmacol.* 1990 Jan 1;39(1):19-26.
59. Franzen CA, Amargo E, Todorović V, et al. The chemopreventive bioflavonoid apigenin inhibits prostate cancer cell motility through the focal adhesion kinase/Src signaling mechanism. *Cancer Prev Res (Phila Pa).* 2009 Sep;2(9):830-41.
60. Gallardo-Williams MT, Chapin RE, King PE, et al. Boron supplementation inhibits the growth and local expression of IGF-1 in human prostate adenocarcinoma(LNCaP) tumors in nude mice. *Toxicol Pathol.* 2004 Jan-Feb;32(1):73-8.
61. Galli F, Stabile AM, Betti M, et al. The effect of alpha- and gamma-tocopherol and their carboxyethyl hydroxychroman metabolites on prostate cancer cell proliferation. *Arch Biochem Biophys.* 2004 Mar 1;423(1):97-102.
62. Gann PH, Ma J, Giovannucci E, et al. Lower prostate cancer risk in men with elevated plasma lycopene levels: results of a prospective analysis. *Cancer Res.* 1999;59:1225-30.
63. Garland CF, Comstock GW, Garland FC, et al. Serum 25-hydroxyvitamin D and colon cancer: eight-year prospective study. *Lancet.* 1989 Nov 18;2(8673):1176-8.
64. Garland CF, Garland FC, Gorham ED. Can colon cancer incidence and death rates be reduced with calcium and vitamin D? *Am J Clin Nutr.* 1991 Jul;54(1 Suppl):193S-201S.
65. Garland CF, Gorham ED, Mohr SB, et al. Vitamin D and prevention of breast cancer: pooled analysis. *J Steroid Biochem Mol Biol.* 2007 Mar;103(3-5):708-11.

66. Gasmi J, Sanderson JT. Growth inhibitory, antiandrogenic, and pro-apoptotic effects of punicic acid in LNCaP human prostate cancer cells. J Agric Food Chem 2010 Nov 10

67. Gerber GS. Phytotherapy for benign prostatic hyperplasia. *Curr Urol Rep.* 2002 Aug;3(4):285-91.

68. Giovannucci E, Ascherio A, Rimm EB, et al. Intake of carotenoids and retinol in relation to risk of prostate cancer. *J Natl Cancer Inst.* 1995;87:1767-76.

69. Glinsky VV, Raz A. Modified citrus pectin anti-metastatic properties: one bullet, multiple targets. *Carbohydr Res.* 2009 Sep 28;344(14):1788-91.

70. Goldmann WH, Sharma AL, Currier SJ, Johnston PD, Rana A, Sharma CP. Saw palmetto berry extract inhibits cell growth and Cox-2 expression in prostatic cancer cells. *Cell Biol Int.* 2001;25(11):1117-24.

71. Gómez Y, Arocha F, Espinoza F, Fernández D, Vásquez A, Granadillo V. Zinc levels in prostatic fluid of patients with prostate pathologies. *Invest Clin.* 2007 Sep;48(3):287-94.

72. Gonzalez A, Peters U, Lampe JW, White E. Zinc intake from supplements and diet and prostate cancer. *Nutr Cancer.* 2009;61(2):206-15.

73. Goodman LA, Jarrett CL, Krunkosky TM, et al. 5-Lipoxygenase expression in benign and malignant canine prostate tissues. *Vet Comp Oncol.* 2011 Jun;9(2):149-57.

74. Gorham ED, Garland CF, Garland FC, et al. Vitamin D and prevention of colorectal cancer. *J Steroid Biochem Mol Biol.* 2005 Oct;97(1-2):179-94.

75. Guess BW, Scholz MC, Strum SB, Lam RY, Johnson HJ, Jennrich RI. Modified citrus pectin (MCP) increases the prostate-specific antigen doubling time in men with prostate cancer: a phase II pilot study. *Prostate Cancer Prostatic Dis.* 2003;6(4):301-4.

76. Gukovsky I, Reyes CN, Vaquero EC, Gukovskaya AS, Pandol SJ. Curcumin ameliorates ethanol and nonethanol experimental pancreatitis. *Am J Physiol Gastrointest Liver Physiol.* 2003 Jan;284(1):G85-95.

77. Gysin R, Azzi A, Visarius T. Gamma-tocopherol inhibits human cancer cell cycle progression and cell proliferation by down-regulation of cyclins. *FASEB J.* 2002 Dec;16(14):1952-4.

78. Haber D. Roads leading to breast cancer. *N Engl J Med.* 2000 Nov 23;343(21):1566-8.

79. Harvei S. Epidemiology of prostatic cancer. *Tidsskr Nor Laegeforen* 1999 Oct 10;119(24):3589-94.

80. Heald CL, Bolton-Smith C, Ritchie MR, Morton MS, Alexander FE. Phyto-oestrogen intake in Scottish men: use of serum to validate a self-administered food-frequency questionnaire in older men. *Eur J Clin Nutr.* 2006 Jan;60(1):129-35.

81. Heath EI, Heilbrun LK, Li J, et al. A phase I dose-escalation study of oral BR-DIM (BioResponse 3,3'- Diindolylmethane) in castrate-resistant, non-metastatic prostate cancer. *Am J Transl Res.* 2010 Jul 23;2(4):402-11.
82. Heber D. Multitargeted therapy of cancer by ellagitannins. *Cancer Lett.* 2008 Oct 8;269(2):262-8.
83. Hedelin M, Klint A, Chang ET, et al. Dietary phytoestrogen, serum enterolactone and risk of prostate cancer: the cancer prostate Sweden study (Sweden). *Cancer Causes Control.* 2006 Mar;17(2):169-80.
84. Helzlsouer KJ, Huang HY, Alberg AJ, et al. Association between alpha-tocopherol, gamma-tocopherol, selenium, and subsequent prostate cancer. *J Natl Cancer Inst.* 2000 Dec 20;92(24):2018-23.
85. Helzlsouer KJ, Huang, HY, Alberg AJ, et al. Association between alpha-tocopherol, gamma-tocopherol, selenium, and subsequent prostate cancer. *J Natl Cancer Inst.* 2000;92:2018-23.
86. Henderson K, Stella SL, Kobylewski S, Eckhert CD. Receptor activated Ca(2+) release is inhibited by boric acid in prostate cancer cells. *PLoS One.* 2009;4(6):e6009.
87. Herman JG, Stadelman HL, Roselli CE. Curcumin blocks CCL2-induced adhesion, motility and invasion, in part, through down-regulation of CCL2 expression and proteolytic activity. *Int J Oncol.* 2009 May;34(5):1319-27.
88. Hirvonen T, Virtamo J, Korhonen P, Albanes D, Pietinen P. Flavonol and flavone intake and the risk of cancer in male smokers (Finland). *Cancer Causes Control.* 2001;12:789-96.
89. Hodges S, Hertz N, Lockwood K, Lister R. CoQ10: could it have a role in cancer management? *Biofactors.* 1999;9(2-4):365-70.
90. Holick MF. Vitamin D deficiency. *N Engl J Med.* 2007 Jul 19;357(3):266-81.
91. Hong JH, Ahn KS, Bae E, Jeon SS, Choi HY. The effects of curcumin on the invasiveness of prostate cancer in vitro and in vivo. *Prostate Cancer Prostatic Dis.* 2006;9(2):147-52.
92. Hong MY, Seeram NP, Heber D. Pomegranate polyphenols down-regulate expression of androgen-synthesizing genes in human prostate cancer cells overexpressing the androgen receptor. *J Nutr Biochem.* 2008 Dec;19(12):848-55.
93. Hostanska K, Suter A, Melzer J, Saller R. Evaluation of cell death caused by an ethanolic extract of Serenoae repentis fructus (Prostasan) on human carcinoma cell lines. *Anticancer Res.* 2007 Mar-Apr;27(2):873-81.
94. Hsieh TC, Wu JM. Grape-derived chemo preventive agent resveratrol decreases prostate-specific antigen (PSA) expression in LNCaP cells by an androgen receptor (AR)-independent mechanism. *Anticancer Res.* 2000 Jan-Feb;20(1A):225-8.
95. http://clinicaltrials.gov/show/NCT01538316.
96. http://my.clevelandclinic.org/heart/prevention/nutrition/omega3.aspx.

97. http://ods.od.nih.gov/factsheets/Selenium-HealthProfessional/.
98. http://www.benthamscience.com/open/tompj/articles/V003/SI0001TO
MPJ/36TOMPJ.pdf.
99. http://www.cancer.gov/cancertopics/pdq/cam/coenzymeQ10/patient/Pa
ge2#Section_23.
100. http://www.cancer.org/treatment/treatmentsandsideeffects/complement
aryandalternativemedicine/dietandnutrition/inositol-hexaphosphate.
101. http://www.cancer.org/treatment/treatmentsandsideeffects/complement
aryandalternativemedicine/ dietandnutrition/modified-citrus-pectin.
102. http://www.lef.org/magazine/mag2012/jul2012_Another-Victory-
Against-FDA-Censorship_01.htm
103. http://www.med.miami.edu/news/view.asp?id=403.
104. http://www.mskcc.org/cancer-care/herb/n-acetylcysteine
105. http://www.mskcc.org/cancer-care/herb/resveratrol.
106. http://www.pcf.org/site/c.leJRIROrEpH/b.5802027/k.D271/Prostate_C
ancer_Risk_Factors.htm.
107. http://www.thorne.com/altmedrev/.fulltext/8/3/303.pdf.
http://www.umm.edu/altmed/articles/gamma-linolenic-000305.htm.
108. http://www.webmd.com/vitamins-supplements/ingredientmono-1018-
N-
ACETYL%20CYSTEINE.aspx?activeIngredientId=1018&activeIngre
dientName=N-ACETYL%20CYSTEINE.
109. Huang L, Kirschke CP, Zhang Y. Decreased intracellular zinc in human
tumorigenic prostate epithelial cells: a possible role in prostate cancer
progression. *Cancer Cell Int.* 2006;6:10.
110. Inohara H, Raz A. Effects of natural complex carbohydrate (citrus
pectin) on murine melanoma cell properties related to galectin-3
functions. *Glycoconj J.* 1994 Dec;11(6):527-32.
111. *Int J Cancer.* 2009 Aug 15;125(4):774-82. doi: 10.1002/ijc.24325.
112. Jacobsen BK, Knutsen SF, Fraser GE. Does high soy milk intake
reduce prostate cancer incidence? The Adventist Health Study (United
States). *Cancer Causes Controls.* 1998 Dec;9(6):553-7.
113. Jang M, Cai L, Udeani GO, et al. Cancer chemopreventive activity of
resveratrol, a natural product derived from grapes. *Science.* 1997 Jan
10;275(5297):218-20.
114. Jang M, Pezzuto JM. Cancer chemopreventive activity of resveratrol.
Drugs Exp Clin Res. 1999;25(2-3):65-77.
115. Jiang Q, Wong J, Ames BN. Gamma-tocopherol induces apoptosis in
androgen-responsive LNCaP prostate cancer cells via caspase-
dependent and independent mechanisms. *Ann NY Acad Sci.* 2004
Dec;1031:399-400.
116. Johansson C, Rytter E, Nygren J, Vessby B, Basu S, Möller L. Down-
regulation of oxidative DNA lesions in human mononuclear cells after
antioxidant supplementation correlates to increase of gamma-
tocopherol. *Int J Vitam Nutr Res.* 2008 Jul-Sep;78(4-5):183-94.

117. Jolliet P, Simon N, Barre J, et al. Plasma coenzyme Q10 concentrations in breast cancer: prognosis and therapeutic consequences. *Int J Clin Pharmacol Ther.* 1998 Sep;36(9):506-9.

118. Kaefer CM, Milner JA. Herbs and Spices in Cancer Prevention and Treatment. In: Benzie IFF, Wachtel-Galor S, editors. Herbal Medicine: Biomolecular and Clinical Aspects. 2nd edition. Boca Raton (FL): CRC Press; 2011.

119. Kampa M, Hatzoglou A, Notas G, et al. Wine antioxidant polyphenols inhibit the proliferation of human prostate cancer cell lines. *Nutr Cancer.* 2000;37(2):223-33.

120. Karna P, Chagani S, Gundala SR, et al. Benefits of whole ginger extract in prostate cancer. *Br J Nutr.* 2012 February;107(4):473-84.

121. Katiyar SK. Matrix metalloproteinases in cancer metastasis: molecular targets for prostate cancer prevention by green tea polyphenols and grape seed proanthocyanidins. *Endocr Metab Immune Disord Drug Targets.* 2006 Mar;6(1):17-24.

122. Kaur M, Agarwal C, Agarwal R. Anticancer and cancer chemopreventive potential of grape seed extract and other grape-based products. *J Nutr.* 2009 Sep;139(9):1806S-12S

123. Khan N, Adhami VM, Mukhtar H. Apoptosis by dietary agents for prevention and treatment of prostate cancer. *Endocr Relat Cancer.* 2010 Mar;17(1):R39-52.

124. Kim J, Jayaprakasha GK, Patil . Limonoids and their anti-proliferative and anti-aromatase properties in human breast cancer cells. BS.*Food Funct.* 2013 Feb;4(2):258-65. doi: 10.1039/c2fo30209h.

125. Kristal AR, Lampe JW. Brassica vegetables and prostate cancer risk: a review of the epidemiological evidence. *Nutr Cancer.* 2002;42(1):1-9.

126. Kucuk O, Sarkar FH, Sakr W, et al. Phase II randomized clinical trial of lycopene supplementation before radical prostatectomy. *Cancer Epidemiol Biomarkers Prev.* 2001;10:861-8.

127. Kunnumakkara AB, Anand P, Aggarwal BB. Curcumin inhibits proliferation, invasion, angiogenesis and metastasis of different cancers through interaction with multiple cell signaling proteins. *Cancer Lett.* 2008 Oct 8;269(2):199-225.

128. Kwon SH[1], Park HY, Kim JY, Jeong IY, Lee MK, Seo KI. Apoptotic action of ursolic acid isolated from Corni fructus in RC-58T/h/SA#4 primary human prostate cancer cells. *Bioorg Med Chem Lett.* 2010 Nov 15;20(22):6435-8. doi: 10.1016/j.bmcl.2010.09.073. Epub 2010 Sep 17.

129. Lalithakumari K, Krishnaraju AV, Sengupta K, Subbaraju GV, Chatterjee A. Safety and toxicological evaluation of a novel, standardized 3-O-acetyl-11-keto-beta-boswellic acid (AKBA)-enriched *Boswellia serrata* extract (5-Loxin(R)). *Toxicol Mech Methods.* 2006;16(4):199-226.

130. Lamblin F, Hano C, Fliniaux O, Mesnard F, Fliniaux MA, Lainé E. Interest of lignans in prevention and treatment of cancers. *Med Sci (Paris).* 2008 May;24(5):511-9.

131. Lansky EP, Newman RA. Punica granatum (pomegranate) and its potential for prevention and treatment of inflammation and cancer. *J Ethnopharmacol*. 2007;109(2):177-206.

132. Lasalvia-Prisco E, Cucchi S, Vazquez J, Lasalvia-Galante E, Golomar W, Gordon W. Serum markers variation consistent with autoschizis induced by ascorbic acid-menadione in patients with prostate cancer. *Med Oncol*. 2003;20(1):45-52.

133. Lee EH, Myung SK, Jeon YJ, et al. Effects of selenium supplements on cancer prevention: Meta-analysis of randomized controlled trials. *Nutr Cancer*. 2011 Nov;63(8):1185-95.

134. Lee MM, Gomez SL, Chang JS, Wey M, Wang RT, Hsing AW. Soy and isoflavone consumption in relation to prostate cancer risk in China. *Cancer Epidemiol Biomarkers Prev*. 2003 Jul;12(7):665-8.

135. Lee YJ, Lee DM, Lee CH, et al. Suppression of human prostate cancer PC-3 cell growth by N-acetylcysteine involves over-expression of Cyr61. *Toxicol In Vitro*. 2011 Feb;25(1):199-205.

136. Lhoste EF, Gloux K, De W, I, et al. The activities of several detoxication enzymes are differentially induced by juices of garden cress, water cress and mustard in human HepG2 cells. *Chem Biol Interact*. 2004 Dec 7;150(3):211-9.

137. Li Y, Chinni SR, Sarkar FH. Selective growth regulatory and pro-apoptotic effects of DIM is mediated by AKT and NF-kappaB pathways in prostate cancer cells. *Front Biosci*. 2005 Jan 1;10:236-43.

138. Li Y, Chinni SR, Sarkar FH. Selective growth regulatory and pro-apoptotic effects of DIM is mediated by AKT and NF-kappaB pathways in prostate cancer cells. *Front Biosci*. 2005 Jan 1;10: 236-43.

139. Liang JY, Liu YY, Zou J, Franklin RB, Costello LC, Feng P. Inhibitory effect of zinc on human prostatic carcinoma cell growth. *Prostate*. 1999;40(3):200-7.

140. Lippman SM, Klein EA, Goodman PJ, et al. Effect of selenium and vitamin E on risk of prostate cancer and other cancers: the Selenium and Vitamin E Cancer Prevention Trial (SELECT). *JAMA*. 2009 Jan 7;301(1):39-51.

141. Liu J-J, Nilsson A, Oredsson S, Badmaev V, Zhao W, Duan R. Boswellic acids trigger apoptosis via a pathway dependent on caspase-8 activation but independent on Fas/Fas ligand interaction in colon cancer HT-29 cells. *Carcinogenesis*. Dec 2002;23(12):2087-93.

142. Liu KC, Yen CY, Wu RS, et al. The roles of endoplasmic reticulum stress and mitochondrial apoptotic signaling pathway in quercetin-mediated cell death of human prostate cancer PC-3 cells. *Environ Toxicol*. 2012. doi: 10.1002/tox.21769. Epub March 20, 2012.

143. Lockwood K, Moesgaard S, Hanioka T, Folkers K. Apparent partial remission of breast cancer in 'high risk' patients supplemented with nutritional antioxidants, essential fatty acids and coenzyme Q10. *Mol Aspects Med*. 1994;15 Suppls231-s40.

144. Lowe JF, Frazee LA. Update on prostate cancer chemoprevention. *Pharmacotherapy.* 2006 Mar;26(3):353-9.

145. Lu QY, Hung JC, Heber D, et al. Inverse associations between plasma lycopene and other carotenoids and prostate cancer. *Cancer Epidemiol Biomarkers Prev.* 2001 Jul;10(7):749-56.

146. Lu R, Serrero G. Resveratrol, a natural product derived from grape, exhibits anti-estrogenic activity and inhibits the growth of human breast cancer cells. *J Cell Physiol.* 1999 Jun;179(3):297-304.

147. Lunoe K, Gabel-Jensen C, Sturup S, Andresen L, Skov S, Gammelgaard B. Investigation of the selenium metabolism in cancer cell lines. *Metallomics.* 2011 Feb;3(2):162-8.

148. Luo H, Jiang BH, King SM, Chen YC. Inhibition of cell growth and VEGF expression in ovarian cancer cells by flavonoids. *Nutr Cancer.* 2008;60(6):800-9.

149. Malik A, Afaq F, Sarfaraz S, Adhami VM, Syed DN, Mukhtar H. Pomegranate fruit juice for chemoprevention and chemotherapy of prostate cancer. *Proc Natl Acad Sci USA.* 2005 Oct 11;102(41):14813-8.

150. Marit Kolberg, Sigrid Pedersen, Nasser E. Bastani, Harald Carlsen, Rune Blomhoff and Ingvild Paur. Tomato Paste Alters NF-κB and Cancer-Related mRNA Expression in Prostate Cancer Cells, Xenografts, and Xenograft Microenvironment. Nutrition and Cancer, Volume 67, Issue 2, 2015, pages 305- 315

151. Marshall JR, Ip C, Romano K, et al. Methyl Selenocysteine: single-dose pharmacokinetics in men. *Cancer Prev Res (Phila).* 2011 Nov;4(11):1938-44.

152. McCann MJ, Gill CI, Linton T, Berrar D, McGlynn H, Rowland IR. Enterolactone restricts the proliferation of the LNCaP human prostate cancer cell line in vitro. *Mol Nutr Food Res.* 2008 May;52(5):567-80.

153. McLarty J, Bigelow RL, Smith M, Elmajian D, Ankem M, Cardelli JA. Tea polyphenols decrease serum levels of prostate-specific antigen, hepatocyte growth factor, and vascular endothelial growth factor in prostate cancer patients and inhibit production of hepatocyte growth factor and vascular endothelial growth factor in vitro. *Cancer Prev Res.* (Phila). 2009 Jul;2(7):673-82.

154. Miano L. Mediterranean diet, micronutrients and prostate carcinoma: a rationale approach to primary prevention of prostate cancer. *Arch Ital Urol Androl.* 2003 Sep;75(3):166-78.

155. Mitchell SH, Zhu W, Young CY. Resveratrol inhibits the expression and function of the androgen receptor in LNCaP prostate cancer cells. *Cancer Res .* 1999 Dec 1;59(23):5892-5.

156. Moyad MA, Brumfield SK, Pienta KJ. Vitamin E, alpha- and gamma-tocopherol, and prostate cancer. *Semin Urol Oncol.* 1999 May;17(2):85-90.

157. Mursu J, Nurmi T, Tuomainen TP, Salonen JT, Pukkala E, Voutilainen S. Intake of flavonoids and risk of cancer in Finnish men: The Kuopio

Ischaemic Heart Disease Risk Factor Study. *Int J Cancer.* 2008;123:660-3.

158. Muti P, Westerlind K, Wu T, et al. Urinary estrogen metabolites and prostate cancer: a case-control study in the United States. *Cancer Causes Control.* 2002 Dec;13(10):947-55.

159. Nair HK, Rao KV, Aalinkeel R, Mahajan S, Chawda R, Schwartz SA. Inhibition of prostate cancer cell colony formation by the flavonoid quercetin correlates with modulation of specific regulatory genes. *Clin Diagn Lab Immunol.* 2004 Jan;11(1):63-9.

160. Nakamura K, Yasunaga Y, Segawa T, et al. Curcumin down-regulates AR gene expression and activation in prostate cancer cell lines. *Int J Oncol.* 2002;21(4):825-30.

161. Nangia-Makker P, Hogan V, Honjo Y, et al. Inhibition of human cancer cell growth and metastasis in nude mice by oral intake of modified citrus pectin. *J Natl Cancer Inst.* 2002 Dec 18;94(24):1854-62.

162. Narayanan BA, Narayanan NK, Re GG, Nixon DW. Differential expression of genes induced by resveratrol in LNCaP cells: P53-mediated molecular targets. *Int J Cancer.* 2003 Mar 20;104(2):204-12.

163. Nassiri-Asl M, Hosseinzadeh H. Review of the pharmacological effects of Vitis vinifera (Grape) and its bioactive compounds. *Phytother Res .* 2009;23:1197-1204.

164. Nimptsch K, Rohrmann S, Linseisen J. Dietary intake of vitamin K and risk of prostate cancer in the Heidelberg cohort of the European Prospective Investigation into Cancer and Nutrition (EPIC-Heidelberg). *Am J Clin Nutr.* 2008 Apr;87(4):985-92.

165. Niture SK, Refai L. Plant pectin: A potential source of cancer suppression. *Amer J Pharmacol Toxicol,* 2013;8(1):9-19.

166. Norrish AE, Skeaff CM, Arribas GL, Sharpe SJ, Jackson RT. Prostate cancer risk and consumption of fish oils: a dietary biomarker-based case-control study. *Br J Cancer.* 1999 Dec;81(7):1238-42.

167. Obermuller-Jevic UC, Olano-Martin E, Corbacho AM, et al. Lycopene inhibits the growth of normal human prostate epithelial cells in vitro. *J Nutr.* 2003;133:3356-60.

168. Ozasa K, Nakao M, Watanabe Y, et al. Serum phytoestrogens and prostate cancer risk in a nested case-control study among Japanese men. *Cancer Sci.* 2004 Jan;95(1):65-71.

169. Pais P. Potency of a novel saw palmetto ethanol extract, SPET-085, for inhibition of 5alpha-reductase II. *Adv Ther.* 2010 Aug;27(8):555-63.

170. Palaniswamy UR, McAvoy RJ, Bible BB, Stuart JD. Ontogenic variations of ascorbic acid and phenethyl isothiocyanate concentrations in watercress (Nasturtium officinale R.Br.) leaves. *J Agric Food Chem.* 2003 Aug 27;51(18):5504-9.

171. Pantuck AJ, et al. Phase II study of pomegranate juice for men with rising prostate-specific antigen following surgery or radiation for prostate cancer. Clin Cancer Res 2006; 12:4018-26

172. Pardee AB, Li YZ, Li CJ. Cancer therapy with beta-lapachone.. *Curr Cancer Drug Targets*. 2002 Sep;2(3):227-42. Review.

173. Perumal SS, Shanthi P, Sachdanandam P. Energy-modulating vitamins—a new combinatorial therapy prevents cancer cachexia in rat mammary carcinoma. *Br J Nutr*. 2005 Jun;93(6):901-9.

174. Pham H, Ziboh VA. 5a-Reductase-catalyzed conversion of testosterone to dihydrotestosterone is increased in prostatic adenocarcinoma cells: suppression by 15-lipoxygenase metabolites of gamma-linolenic and eicosapentaenoic acids. *Steroid Biochem Mol Biol*. 2002;82:393-400.

175. Pienta KJ, Naik H, Akhtar A, et al. Inhibition of spontaneous metastasis in a rat prostate cancer model by oral administration of modified citrus pectin. *J Natl Cancer Inst*. 1995;87:348-53.

176. Pietinen P, Stumpf K, Männistö S, Kataja V, Uusitupa M, Adlercreutz H. Serum enterolactone and risk of breast cancer: a case-control study in eastern Finland. *Cancer Epidemiol Biomarkers Prev*. 2001 Apr;10(4):339-44.

177. Piller R, Chang-Claude J, Linseisen J. Plasma enterolactone and genistein and the risk of premenopausal breast cancer. *Eur J Cancer Prev*. 2006 Jun;15(3):225-32.

178. Plummer SM, Holloway KA, Manson MM, et al. Inhibition of cyclo-oxygenase 2 expression in colon cells by the chemopreventive agent curcumin involves inhibition of NF-kappaB activation via the NIK/IKK signalling complex. *Oncogene*. 1999 Oct 28;18(44):6013-20.

179. Polesel J, Talamini R, Montella M, et al. Linoleic acid, vitamin D and other nutrient intakes in the risk of non-Hodgkin lymphoma: an Italian case-control study. *Ann Oncol*. 2006 Apr;17(4):713-8.

180. Pomegranate ellagitannin-derived metabolites inhibit prostate cancer growth and localize to the mouse prostate gland. Seeram NP[1], Aronson WJ, Zhang Y, Henning SM, Moro A, Lee RP, Sartippour M, Harris DM, Rettig M, Suchard MA, Pantuck AJ, Belldegrun A, Heber D. J Agric Food Chem. 2007 Sep 19;55(19):7732-7. Epub 2007 Aug 28.

181. Portakal O, Ozkaya O, Erden IM, et al. Coenzyme Q10 concentrations and antioxidant status in tissues of breast cancer patients. *Clin Biochem*. 2000 Jun;33(4): 279-84.

182. Prins GS, Tang WY, Belmonte J, Ho SM. Perinatal exposure to oestradiol and bisphenol A alters the prostate epigenome and increases susceptibility to carcinogenesis. *Basic Clin Pharmacol Toxicol*. 2008 Feb;102(2):134-8.

183. Rafi MM, Kanakasabai S, Reyes MD, Bright JJ. Lycopene modulates growth and survival associated genes in prostate cancer. J Nutr Biochem. 2013 Oct;24(10):1724-34.

184. Raina K, Ravichandran K, Rajamanickam S, Huber KM, Serkova NJ, Agarwal R. Inositol hexaphosphate inhibits tumor growth, vascularity, and metabolism in TRAMP mice: a multiparametric magnetic resonance study. *Cancer Prev Res*. January 2013;6:40-50.

185. Raina K, Singh RP, Agarwal R, Agarwal C. Oral grape seed extract inhibits prostate tumor growth and progression in TRAMP mice. *Cancer Res.* 2007;67:5976-82.

186. Rajashekhar G, Willuweit A, Patterson CE, et al. Continuous endothelial cell activation increases angiogenesis: evidence for the direct role of endothelium linking angiogenesis and inflammation. *J Vasc Res.* 2006;43(2):193-204.

187. Reagan-Shaw S, Nihal M, Ahmad N. Dose translation from animal to human studies revisited. *FASEB J.* 2008;22:659-61.

188. Ren S, Lien EJ. Natural products and their derivatives as cancer chemopreventive agents. *Prog Drug Res.* 1997;48:147-71.

189. Rusciani L, Proietti I, Rusciani A, et al. Low plasma coenzyme Q10 levels as an independent prognostic factor for melanoma progression. *J Am Acad Dermatol.* 2006 Feb;54(2):234-41.

190. Safayhi H, Rall B, Sailer ER, Ammon HP. Inhibition by boswellic acids of human leukocyte elastase. *J Pharmacol Exp T*her. 1997 Apr;281(1):460-3.

191. Safayhi H, Sailer ER, Ammon HP. Mechanism of 5-lipoxygenase inhibition by acetyl-11-keto-beta-boswellic acid. *Mol Pharmacol.* 1995 Jun;47(6):1212-6.

192. Sakr WA, Grignon DJ, Haas GP, et al. Epidemiology of high grade prostatic intraepithelial neoplasia. *Pathol Res Pract.* 1995 Sep;191(9):838-41.

193. Sampson AP. FLAP inhibitors for the treatment of inflammatory diseases. *Curr Opin Investig Drugs.* 2009 Nov;10(11):1163-72.

194. Sarkar FH, Li Y. Indole-3-carbinol and prostate cancer. *J Nutr.* 2004 Dec;134(12 Suppl):3493S-3498S.

195. Sartippour MR et al. Ellagitannin-rich pomegranate extract inhibits angiogenesis in prostate cancer in vitro and in vivo. Intl J Oncol 2008; 32:475-80

196. Schleicher RL, Lamartiniere CA, Zheng M, et al. The inhibitory effect of genistein on the growth and metastasis of a transplantable rat accessory sex gland carcinoma. *Cancer Lett.* 1999 Mar 1;136(2):195-201.

197. Seeni A, Takahashi S, Takeshita K, et al. Suppression of prostate cancer growth by resveratrol in the transgenic rat for adenocarcinoma of prostate (TRAP) model. *Asian Pac J Cancer Prev.* 2008 Jan-Mar;9(1):7-14.

198. Seeram NP et al. In vitro antiproliferative, apoptotic and antioxidant activities of punicalagin, ellagic acid and a total pomegranate tannin extract are enhanced in combination with other polyphenols as found in pomegranate juice. J Nutr Biochem 2005 Jun; 16(6):360-67.

199. Senthilkumar K, Arunkumar R, Elumalai P, et al. Quercetin inhibits invasion, migration and signalling molecules involved in cell survival and proliferation of prostate cancer cell line (PC-3). *Cell Biochem Funct.* 2011 Mar;29(2):87-95.

200. Shabbeer S1, Sobolewski M, Anchoori RK, Kachhap S, Hidalgo M, Jimeno A, Davidson N, Carducci MA, Khan SR. Fenugreek: a naturally occurring edible spice as an anticancer agent. *Cancer Biol Ther*. 2009 Feb;8(3):272-8. Epub 2009 Feb 18.

201. Shamsuddin AM, Yang GY. Inositol hexaphosphate inhibits growth and induces differentiation of PC-3 human prostate cancer cells. *Carcinogenesis*. 1995 Aug;16(8):1975-9.

202. Shen JC, Klein RD, Wei Q, et al. Low-dose genistein induces cyclin-dependent kinase inhibitors and G(1) cell-cycle arrest in human prostate cancer cells. *Mol Carcinog*. 2000 Oct;29(2):92-102.

203. Shi Q, Shih CC, Lee KH. Novel anti-prostate cancer curcumin analogues that enhance androgen receptor degradation activity. *Anticancer Agents Med Chem*. 2009 Oct;9(8):904-12.

204. Shishodia S, Chaturvedi MM, Aggarwal BB. Role of curcumin in cancer therapy. *Curr Probl Cancer*. 2007 Jul-Aug;31(4):243-305.

205. Shui IM, Mucci LA, Kraft P, et al. Vitamin D-related genetic variation, plasma vitamin D, and risk of lethal prostate cancer: a prospective nested case-control study. *J Natl Cancer Inst*. 2012 May 2;104(9):690-9.

206. Shukla S, Gupta S. Apigenin: A promising molecule for cancer prevention. *Pharm Res*. 2010 June;27(6):962-78.

207. Shukla S, Mishra A, Fu P, Maclennan GT, Resnick MI, Gupta S. Up-regulation of insulin-like growth factor binding protein-3 by apigenin leads to growth inhibition and apoptosis of 22Rv1 xenograft in athymic nude mice. *FASEB J*. 2005 Dec;19(14):2042-44.

208. Shukla Y, Singh M. Cancer preventive properties of ginger: a brief review. *Food Chem Toxicol*. 2007 May;45(5):683-90.

209. Siegel R, Naishadham D, Jemal A. Cancer statistics 2012. *CA Cancer J Clin*. 2012;62:10-29.

210. Sineh Sepehr K, Baradaran B, Mazandarani M, Khori V, Shahneh FZ. Studies on the cytotoxic activities of Punica granatum L. var. spinosa (Apple Punice) extract on prostate cell line by induction of apoptosis. *ISRN Pharm*. 2012;2012:547942.

211. Singh RP, Agarwal R. A cancer chemopreventive agent silibinin, targets mitogenic and survival signaling in prostate cancer. *Mutat Res*. 2004 Nov 2;555(1-2):21-32.

212. Singh RP, Agarwal R. Prostate cancer prevention by silibinin. *Curr Cancer Drug Targets*. 2004 Feb;4(1):1-11.

213. Singh RP, Sharma G, Dhanalakshmi S, Agarwal C, Agarwal R. Suppression of advanced human prostate tumor growth in athymic mice by silibinin feeding is associated with reduced cell proliferation, increased apoptosis, and inhibition of angiogenesis. *Cancer Epidemiol Biomarkers Prev*. 2003 Sept;12(9):933-9.

214. Singh RP, Sharma G, Mallikarjuna GU, Dhanalakshmi S, Agarwal C, Agarwal R. In vivo suppression of hormone-refractory prostate cancer growth by inositol hexaphosphate: induction of insulin-like growth

factor binding protein-3 and inhibition of vascular endothelial growth factor. *Clin Cancer Res.* 2004 Jan 1;10(1 Pt 1):244-50.

215. Sirab N, Robert G, Fasolo V, et al. Lipidosterolic extract of serenoa repens modulates the expression of inflammation related-genes in benign prostatic hyperplasia epithelial and stromal cells. *Int J Mol Sci.* 2013 Jul 10;14(7):14301-20.

216. Skinner HG, Michaud DS, Giovannucci E, et al. Vitamin D intake and the risk for pancreatic cancer in two cohort studies. *Cancer Epidemiol Biomarkers Prev.* 2006 Sep;15(9):1688-95.

217. Soares ND, Teodoro AJ, Oliveira FL, et al. Influence of lycopene on cell viability, cell cycle, and apoptosis of human prostate cancer and benign hyperplastic cells. Nutr Cancer. 2013 Sep 20.

218. Sonoda T, Nagata Y, Mori M, et al. A case-control study of diet and prostate cancer in Japan: possible protective effect of traditional Japanese diet. *Cancer Sci.* 2004 Mar;95(3):238-42.

219. Stark A, Madar Z. Phytoestrogens: a review of recent findings. *J Pediatr Endocrinol Metab.* 2002 May;15(5):561-72.

220. Steiner MS, Raghow S. Antiestrogens and selective estrogen receptor modulators reduce prostate cancer risk. *World J Urol.* 2003 May;21(1):31-6.

221. Stone WL, Papas AM. Tocopherols and the etiology of colon cancer. *J Natl Cancer Inst.* 1997 Jul 16;89(14):1006-14.

222. Supabphol A, Supabphol R. Antimetastatic potential of N-acetylcysteine on human prostate cancer cells. *J Med Assoc Thai.* 2012 Dec;95 Suppl 12:S56-62.

223. Sutcliffe S, Giovannucci E, Leitzmann MF, Rimm EB, Stampfer MJ, et al. A prospective cohort study of red wine consumption and risk of prostate cancer. *Int J Cancer.* 2007;120:1529-35.

224. Suzuki M, Endo M, Shinohara F, Echigo S, Rikiishi H. Differential apoptotic response of human cancer cells to organoselenium compounds. *Cancer Chemother Pharmacol.* 2010 Aug;66(3):475-84.

225. Suzuki R, Rylander-Rudqvist T, Saji S, Bergkvist L, Adlercreutz H, Wolk A. Dietary lignans and postmenopausal breast cancer risk by oestrogen receptor status: a prospective cohort study of Swedish women. *Br J Cancer.* 2008 Feb 12;98(3):636-40.

226. Takase Y, Levesque MH, Luu-The V, et al. Expression of enzymes involved in estrogen metabolism in human prostate. *J Histochem Cytochem.* 2006 Aug;54(8):911-21.

227. Tareen B, Summers JL, Jamison JM, et al. A 12 week, open label, phase I/IIa study using apatone for the treatment of prostate cancer patients who have failed standard therapy. *Int J Med Sci.* 2008;5(2):62-7.

228. Teiten MH, Gaascht F, Eifes S, Dicato M, Diederich M. Chemopreventive potential of curcumin in prostate cancer. *Genes Nutr.* 2010 Mar;5(1):61-74.

229. Thirugnanam S, Xu L, Ramaswamy K, Gnanasekar M. Glycyrrhizin induces apoptosis in prostate cancer cell lines DU-145 and LNCaP. *Oncol Rep.* 2008 Dec;20(6):1387-92.

230. Thomas RJ, Williams MMA, Sharma H, et al. A double-blind, placebo RCT evaluating the effect of a polyphenol-rich whole food supplement on PSA progression in men with prostate cancer: The U.K. National Cancer Research Network (NCRN) Pomi-T study. *J Clin Oncol.* 2013;31(suppl):abstract 5008.

231. Toit-Kohn JL, Louw L, Engelbrecht. Docosahexaenoic acid induces apoptosis in colorectal carcinoma cells by modulating the PI3 kinase and p38 MAPK pathways. AM. J Nutr Biochem. 2009 Feb;20(2):106-14. doi: 10.1016/*j.jnutbio.*2007.12.005. Epub 2008 May 13.

232. Trejo-Solís C, Pedraza-Chaverrí J, Torres-Ramos M, et al. Multiple molecular and cellular mechanisms of action of lycopene in cancer inhibition. *Evid Based Complement Alternat Med.* 2013;2013:705121.

233. Tsui KH, Feng TH, Lin CM, Chang PL, Juang HH. Curcumin blocks the activation of androgen and interlukin-6 on prostate-specific antigen expression in human prostatic carcinoma cells. *J Androl.* 2008 Nov-Dec;29(6):661-8.

234. USDA. Available at: http://www.isoflavones.info/isoflavones-content.php. Accessed September 9, 2013.

235. Vayalil PK, Mittal A, Katiyar SK. Proanthocyanidins from grape seeds inhibit expression of matrix metalloproteinases in human prostate carcinoma cells, which is associated with the inhibition of activation of MAPK and NF kappa B. *Carcinogenesis.* 2004;25:987-95.

236. Venkateswaran, V, Klotz, LH, Fleshner, NE. Selenium modulation of cell proliferation and cell cycle biomarkers in human prostate carcinoma cell lines. *Cancer Res.* 2002;62:2540-5. Klein EA, Thompson IM, Jr., Tangen CM, et al. Vitamin E and the risk of prostate cancer: the Selenium and Vitamin E Cancer Prevention Trial (SELECT). *JAMA.* 2011 Oct 12;306(14):1549-56.

237. von Holtz RL, Fink CS, Awad AB. Beta-Sitosterol activates the sphingomyelin cycle and induces apoptosis in LNCaP human prostate cancer cells. *Nutr Cancer.* 1998;32(1):8-12.

238. Vucenik I[1], Shamsuddin AM. Protection against cancer by dietary IP6 and inositol. *Nutr Cancer.* 2006;55(2):109-25..

239. Wang LQ. Mammalian phytoestrogens: enterodiol and enterolactone. *J Chromatogr B Analyt Technol Biomed Life Sci.* 2002 Sep 25;777(1-2):289-309.

240. *Hsing AW, Comstock GW, Abbey H, Polk BF. Serologic precursors of cancer. Retinol, carotenoids, and tocopherol and risk of prostate cancer.J Natl Cancer Inst 1990;82:941-6.* (70)↵

241. *Gann PH, Ma J, Giovannucci E, Willett W, Sacks F, Hennekens CH, et al. A prospective analysis of plasma antioxidants and prostate cancer risk [abstract]. Proc Am Assoc Cancer Res 1998;39:89.* (71)↵

242. *Nomura AM, Stemmermann GN, Lee J, Craft NE. Serum micronutrients and prostate cancer in Japanese Americans in Hawaii. Cancer Epidemiol Biomarkers Prev 1997;6:487-91.*

Flax seed references

243. In a recent French study conducted over 7 years with 58,049 women participants concluded….. "High dietary intakes of plant lignans were associated with reduced risks of breast cancer in a Western population that does not consume a diet rich in soy".Published Journal National Cancer Institute 2007;99:475-86. Touilland, Thiebout, et al.

244. "Cancers of the breast and prostate, in their early phase of development, are hormone dependant and could be influenced by endocrine changes induced by lignans". Morton MS Wilcox G Wahlqvist ML Griffiths KDetermination of lignans and isoflavonoids in human female plasma following dietary supplementation

245. Dietary estrogens, such as lignan-rich flaxseed, are similar in structure to endogenous sex steroid hormones and act in vivo to alter hormone metabolism and reduce subsequent cancer risk in postmenopausal women.(Hutchins A, Cancer Epidemiol Biomarkers Prev, 9(10): 1113, 2000)

246. There is considerable evidence from epidemiological studies correlating high concentrations of lignans in the body fluids with a low incidence of hormone-dependent tumors, in particular breast cancer. Kulling SE Jacobs E Pfeiffer E Metzler MStudies on the genotoxicity of the mammalian lignans enterolactone and enterodiol and their metabolic precursors at various endpoints in vitro. In: Mutat Res (1998 Aug 7) 416(1 2):115 24

247. There is a substantial reduction in breast cancer risk among women with a high intake (as measured by excretion) of phyto-oestrogens - particularly the isoflavonic phyto-oestrogens equol and the lignan enterolactone. These findings could be important in the prevention of breast cancer. Ingram D Sanders K Kolybaba M Lopez D Case control study of phyto oestrogens and breast cancer In: Lancet (1997 Oct 4) 350(9083):990 4

248. Phytoestrogens are diphenolic compounds that are present in several plants eaten by human beings. Flaxseed is a particularly abundant source of phytoestrogens. When ingested in relatively large amounts, phytoestrogens have been shown to have significant estrogen agonists/antagonists effects in animals and humans. There is epidemiological, laboratory and clinical evidence which indicates that phytoestrogens, like certain selective estrogen receptor modulators, have an antiproliferative effect on the breast, and positive effects on the lipoprotein profile and bone density. They might also improve some of the climacteric symptoms.(Brzezinski A & Bebi A. Eur J Obstet Gynecol Reprod Biol. 85(1): 47, 1999

249. Maximum combined concentrations of lignans, during the linseed supplemental period approached 500 ng/ml. This value although representing the total rather than the free fraction, is some 10,000 times the concentration of free oestradiol seen in postmenopausal women and similar to the levels of the anti-estrogen Tamoxifin observed with breast cancer treated with 20 mg/day of this drug.

250. Morton MS Wilcox G Wahlqvist ML Griffiths K Determination of lignans and isoflavonoids in human female plasma following dietary supplementation.

251. Flaxseed is high in secoisolariciresinol diglycoside (SDG), the precursor of mammalian lignans, which can affect mammary gland structure. Lifetime or gestation and lactation exposure to 5 or 10% flaxseed induce structural changes in the mammary gland that may potentially reduce mammary cancer risk.(Tou J & Thompson L. Carcinogenesis, 20(9): 1831, 1999)

252. Flaxseed and SDG, regardless of dose, appeared to delay the progression of MNU-induced mammary tumorigenesis. (Rickard S. et al, Nutr Cancer; 35(1): 50, 1999)

253. Dietary supplementation with secoisolariciresinol diglycoside (SDG), a lignan precursor isolated from flaxseed, significantly reduced pulmonary metastasis cells and inhibited the growth of metastatic tumors that formed in the lungs. (Li D. et al, Cancer Lett, 142(1): 91, 1999)

254. Flaxseed the richest source of lignans reduces metastasis and inhibits the growth of the metastatic secondary tumors in animals. Flaxseed may be a useful nutritional adjuvant to prevent melanoma metastasis in cancer patients.(Yan L, et al, Cancer Lett, 124(2): 181, 1998)

255. The mammalian lignans enterolactone (EL) and enterodiol (ED) derived from precursors in foods, particularly flaxseed, have been shown to reduce the mammary tumor growth due to their antiestrogenic properties. Lignans are growth inhibitors of colon tumor cells and they may act through mechanism(s) other than antiestrogenic activity.(Sung M, et al, Anticancer Res 18(3A: 1405, 1998)

256. Excretion of both equol and enterolactone was associated with a substantial reduction in breast-cancer risk, with significant trends. Ingram D Sanders K Kolybaba M Lopez D Case control study of phyto oestrogens and breast cancer In: Lancet (1997 Oct 4) 350(9083):990 4

257. Mammalian lignans inhibit the growth of human breast cancer cells and partially inhibit angiogenesis. Rickard SE Orcheson LJ Seidl MM Luyengi L Fong HH Thompson LUDose dependent production of mammalian lignans in rats and in vitro from the purified precursor secoisolaricire

258. Epidemiological studies indicated that plasma levels and urinary excretion of the lignan and isoflavonoid phytoestrogens correlated negatively with rates of breast and prostate cancer. Ren S Lien EJ Natural products and their derivatives as cancer

259. The lignan enterolactone showed a three-fold reduction (reduction in risk for breast cancer) in risk for the highest compared with the lowest quartile of excretion... Ingram D Sanders K Kolybaba M Lopez DCase control study of phyto oestrogens and breast cancer In: Lancet (1997 Oct 4) 350(9083):990 4

260. Many Lignans have antitumor, antimitotic, antioxidant, weak estrogenic and antiestrogenic activities and some have been shown to prevent the growth of many tumors studied in the chemotherapy program of the U.S. National Cancer Institute. Mammalian Lignan Production From Various Foods Nutrition and Cancer; Lawrence Erlbaum Associates, Inc. 1991

261. Flax is a potent source of lignans.... studies suggested that they may interfere with the development of breast, prostate, colon, and other tumors in humans. Journal of the National Cancer Institute. Vol. 86 No.23. December 7, 1994 pg. 1748

262. They (lignans) have now been shown to influence not only sex-hormone metabolism and biological activity but also intracellular enzymes, protein synthesis, growth factor action, malignant cell proliferation, differentiation and angiogenesis, making them strong candidates as natural cancer chemo-preventative compounds. Ren S Lien EJNatural products and their derivatives as cancer chemopreventive agents. In: Prog Drug Res (1997) 48:147 71

263. A great deal of evidence supports the hypothesis that adequate lignan and isoflavone intakes reduce cancer risk. Several papers have reviewed the potential roles of phytoestrogens in preventing breast, colon, and prostate cancer. Kurzer MS Xu X Dietary phytoestrogens. In: Annu Rev Nutr (1997) 17:353 81

264. In addition to their inhibition of malignant cell proliferation the lignans may be protective with regard to PC (prostate cancer) or benign prostatic hyperplasia (BPH) due to their moderate aromatase inhibiting activity or to an effect on free testosterone levels via inhibition of LH secretion stimulation of SHBG synthesis. Both group of phytoestrogens show antioxidant properties which may play a role in carcinogenesis.

265. Aldercreutz H Makela S Pylkkanen L Santti R Kinzel J van Reijsen M Markkanen H Kamarainen EL Watanabe S Fotsis T et alDietary phytoestrogens and prostate cancer (Meeting abstract).

266. Flaxseed, a rich source of mammalian lignan precursor secoisolariciresinol-diglucoside (S.D.) And alpha-linolenic acid (ALA) has been shown to be protective at the early promotion stage of carcinogenesis.

267. Thompson LU Rickard SE Orcheson LJ Seidl MMFlaxseed and its lignan and oil components reduce mammary tumor growth at a late stage of carcinogenesis. In: Carcinogenesis (1996 Jun) 17(6):1373 6. Health Effects of Flaxseed Mucilage, Lignans Inform, Vol. 8, no. 8 (August 1997)

268. Higher urinary levels have been found in humans and animals at lower risk of developing cancer. Rickard SE Orcheson LJ Seidl MM Luyengi L Fong HH Thompson LU Dose dependent production of mammalian lignans in rats and in vitro from the puri

269. LeBeau AM, Kostova M, Craik CS, Denmeade SR. Prostate-specific antigen: an overlooked candidate for the targeted treatment and selective imaging of prostate cancer. Biol Chem. 2010 Apr;391(4):333-43.

270. Korkmaz M, Avci CB, Gunduz C, Aygunes D, Erbaykent-Tepedelen B. Disodium pentaborate decahydrate (DPD) induced apoptosis by decreasing hTERT enzyme activity and disrupting F-actin organization of prostate cancer cells. Tumour Biol. 2014 Feb;35(2):1531-8.

271. Zhang Z-F, Winton MI, Rainey C, et al. Boron is associated with decreased risk of human prostate cancer. FASEB J. 2001;15:A1089.

272. Barranco WT, Eckhert CD. Boric acid inhibits human prostate cancer cell proliferation. Cancer Lett. 2004 Dec 8;216(1):21-9.

273. Schaafsma A, de Vries PJ, Saris WH. Delay of natural bone loss by higher intakes of specific minerals and vitamins. Crit Rev Food Sci Nutr. 2001 May;41(4):225-49.

274. Cui Y, Winton MI, Zhang ZF, et al. Dietary boron intake and prostate cancer risk. Oncol Rep. 2004 Apr;11(4):887-92.

275. Gallardo-Williams MT, Chapin RE, King PE, et al. Boron supplementation inhibits the growth and local expression of IGF-1 in human prostate adenocarcinoma (LNCaP) tumors in nude mice. Toxicol Pathol. 2004 Jan-Feb;32(1):73-8.

276. Webber MM, Waghray A, Bello D. Prostate-specific antigen, a serine protease, facilitates human prostate cancer cell invasion. Clin Cancer Res. 1995 Oct;1(10):1089-94.

277. Gallardo-Williams MT, Maronpot RR, Wine RN, et al. Inhibition of the enzymatic activity of prostate-specific antigen by boric acid and 3-nitrophenyl boronic acid. Prostate. 2003 Jan 1;54(1):44-9.

278. Cohen P, Graves HC, Peehl DM, et al. Prostate-specific antigen (PSA) is an insulin-like growth factor binding protein-3 protease found in seminal plasma. J Clin Endocrinol Metab. 1992 Oct;75(4):1046-53.

279. Cohen P, Peehl DM, Graves HC, et al. Biological effects of prostate specific antigen as an insulin-like growth factor binding protein-3 protease. J Endocrinol. 1994 Sep;142(3):407-15.

280. Henderson K, Stella SL, Kobylewski S, Eckhert CD. Receptor activated Ca(2+) release is inhibited by boric acid in prostate cancer cells. PLOS One. 2009;4(6):e6009.

281. Chang SS. Overview of prostate-specific membrane antigen. Rev Urol. 2004;6(Suppl 10):S13-8.

282. El-Zaria ME, Genady AR, Janzen N, Petlura CI, Beckford VDR, Valliant JF. Preparation and evaluation of carborane-derived inhibitors of prostate specific membrane antigen (PSMA). Dalton Trans. 2014 Apr 7;43(13):4950-61.

283. Tombal B, Lecouvet F. Modern detection of prostate cancer's bone metastasis: Is the bone scan era over? Adv Urol. 2012;2012:893193.
284. Available at: http://www.turner-white.com/memberfile.php?PubCode=hp_nov04_bone.pdf. Accessed August 23, 2015.
285. Jimenez-Andrade JM, Mantyh WG, Bloom AP, Ferng AS, Geffre CP, Mantyh PW. Bone cancer pain. Ann N Y Acad Sci. 2010 Jun;1198:173-81.
286. Miggiano GA, Gagliardi L. Diet, nutrition and bone health. Clin Ter. 2005 Jan-Apr;156(1-2):47-56.Nielsen FH, Hunt CD, Mullen LM, Hunt JR. Effect of dietary boron on mineral, estrogen, and testosterone metabolism in postmenopausal women. FASEB J. 1987 Nov;1(5):394-7.
287. Nielsen FH, Hunt CD, Mullen LM, Hunt JR. Effect of dietary boron on mineral, estrogen, and testosterone metabolism in postmenopausal women. FASEB J. 1987 Nov;1(5):394-7.
288. Hegsted M, Keenan MJ, Siver F, Wozniak P. Effect of boron on vitamin D deficient rats. Biol Trace Elem Res. 1991 Mar;28(3):243-55.
289. Scorei ID, Scorei RI. Calcium fructoborate helps control inflammation associated with diminished bone health. Biol Trace Elem Res. 2013 Dec;155(3):315-21.
290. Available at: http://www.cdc.gov/nchs/fastats/arthritis.htm. Accessed August 23, 2015.
291. Naghii MR, Mofid M, Asgari AR, Hedayati M, Daneshpour MS. Comparative effects of daily and weekly boron supplementation on plasma steroid hormones and proinflammatory cytokines. J Trace Elem Med Biol. 2011 Jan;25(1):54-8.
292. Hunt CD, Idso JP. Dietary boron as a physiological regulator of the normal inflammatory response: A review and current research progress. J Trace Elem Exp Med. 1999 Jul 19;12(3):221-33.
293. Travers RL, Rennie GC, Newnham RE: Boron and arthritis: the result of a double-blind pilot study. J Nutr Environ Med. 1990;1(2):127-32.
294. Helliwell TR, Kelly SA, Walsh HP, et al. Elemental analysis of femoral bone from patients with fractured neck of femur or osteoarthrosis. Bone. 1996 Feb;18(2):151-7.
295. Hall IH, Rajendran KG, Chen SY, et al. Anti-inflammatory activity of amine-carboxyboranes in rodents. Arch Pharm (Weinheim). 1995 Jan;328(1):39-44.
296. Rajendran KG, Chen SY, Sood A, Spielvogel BF, Hall IH. The anti-osteoporotic activity of amine-carboxyboranes in rodents. Biomed Pharmacother. 1995;49(3):131-40.
297. Hall IH, Starnes CO, McPhail AT, et al. Anti-inflammatory activity of amine cyanoboranes, amine carboxyboranes, and related compounds. J Pharm Sci . 1980 Sep;69(9):1025-9.
298. Newnham RE. Essentiality of boron for healthy bones and joints. Environ Health Perspect. 1994 Nov;102 Suppl 7:83-5.

299. Available at: http://www.cdc.gov/cancer/prostate/statistics/index.htm. Accessed August 23, 2015.
300. Available at: http://www.cdc.gov/cancer/dcpc/data/men.htm. Accessed August 23, 2015.
301. Available at: http://www.cdc.gov/cancer/prostate/index.htm. Accessed August 23, 2015.
302. Available at: http://www.cdc.gov/cancer/prostate/basic_info/symptoms.htm. Accessed August 23, 2015.
303. Available at: http://www.greenfacts.org/en/boron/toolboxes/2.htm. Accessed August 23, 2015.
304. Available at: http://hypertextbook.com/facts/2009/AliciaMcGeachy.shtml. Accessed August 23, 2015.
305. Rainey C, Nyquist L. Multicountry estimation of dietary boron intake. Biological trace element research. Winter 1998;66(1-3):79-86.
306. Available at: http://www.cancer.gov/types/prostate/hp/prostate-prevention-pdq#section/all. Accessed 8/20/2015.
307. Holund B. Latent prostatic cancer in a consecutive autopsy series. Scand J Urol Nephrol. 1980;14(1):29-35.
308. Sakr WA, Haas GP, Cassin BF et al. The frequency of carcinoma and intraepithelial neoplasia of the prostate in young male patients. J Urol. 1993 Aug;150(2 Pt 1):379-85.

www.ingramcontent.com/pod-product-compliance
Lightning Source LLC
Chambersburg PA
CBHW070321190526
45169CB00005B/1695